# ACLS Quick Review Study Cards

**Barbara Aehlert, RN**
Director, EMS Education and Research
Samaritan Health System
Phoenix, Arizona

Publisher: David T. Culverwell
Executive Editor: Richard A. Weimer
Development Editor: Julie Scardiglia
Editorial Assistant: Kay E. Beard
Book Design and Production: Cynthia Edmiston, Merrifield Graphics & Publishing Service, Inc.
Cover Design: Gillian Johnson



Printed in the United States of America

Mosby-Year Book, Inc.
11830 Westline Industrial Drive
St. Louis, Missouri 63146

# INTRODUCTION

These study cards are designed for use by physicians, nurses, prehospital providers, respiratory therapists and allied health professionals preparing for the American Heart Association's Advanced Cardiac Life Support (ACLS) Provider Course. They may also be used as a review in preparation for the ACLS Instructor Course by those persons identified during the ACLS Provider course as instructor-potential by the Course Director.

These cards supplement the AHA materials and provide a review of the material presented in the ACLS course based on the American Heart Association guidelines published in October 1992.

The material in each section of these study cards is color-coded to correspond with the text – ACLS Quick Review Study Guide (Mosby Lifeline, 1994). The text provides a summary of the core material presented in the ACLS Provider course with a pretest, post-test and quizzes provided for self-evaluation. The ACLS Quick Review Study Cards supplement the text and provide additional review of the core ACLS material through the use of 500 questions and short-answers. A question appears on the front of each card and the correct answer, with accompanying rationale, appears on the back. The cards are labelled according to the subject areas; however, each card is independent of the others, eliminating the need to place the cards is a specific sequence.

These cards may be used independently for individual review or in group study sessions. I hope you find them useful and welcome your comments and suggestions.

Barbara Aehlert, RN

# ACKNOWLEDGMENTS

My thanks to David Culverwell, Publisher, and Richard Weimer, Executive Editor, Mosby Lifeline for believing in the merit of this venture.

I would also like to thank James Haner, CEP, Greg Ruiz, CEP, Marcus Steele, CEP, Mary Alice Witzel, RN, Ernie Cano, John Delaney, Brian Hall, Brian Kotsur, Troy Miller, Garret Olson, Ty Perkins, and Scott Trimble who reviewed portions of these study cards.

Thanks also to Cynthia Edmiston of Merrifield Graphics and Publishing Service, Inc. for the contribution of your talent and hard work to this undertaking; and to Gillian Johnson, also of Merrifield Graphics, for your cover design.

A very special thanks to Julie Scardiglia, Development Editor, Mosby Lifeline. I value your comments, respect your expertise and have sincerely enjoyed working with you on this project.

# DEDICATION

For my father, Bobby R. Mahoney

# CONTENTS

## MYOCARDIAL INFARCTION

Name the primary mechanisms of out-of-hospital cardiac arrest.

## MYOCARDIAL INFARCTION

Administration of prophylactic lidocaine to patients with suspected MI is no longer recommended.

What is meant by the term "prophylactic" lidocaine?

## MYOCARDIAL INFARCTION

Name three signs and symptoms of pulmonary congestion.

## MYOCARDIAL INFARCTION

Define the terms "transmural" and "subendocardial" myocardial infarction.

## MYOCARDIAL INFARCTION

Define "myocardial infarction."

## MYOCARDIAL INFARCTION

Why is pain relief a high priority in the management of acute myocardial infarction?

## MYOCARDIAL INFARCTION

What are the qualifying criteria for administration of thrombolytic therapy in acute myocardial infarction?

## MYOCARDIAL INFARCTION

Why is hypertension potentially harmful in acute myocardial infarction?

## MYOCARDIAL INFARCTION

Prophylactic lidocaine refers to administration of this drug to patients with suspected acute myocardial infarction who do not have ventricular ectopy.

## MYOCARDIAL INFARCTION

The primary mechanisms of out-of-hospital cardiac arrest are:

- Ventricular fibrillation (most common)
- Ventricular tachycardia
- Bradydysrhythmias
  - including asystole and pulseless electrical activity
- Supraventricular tachydysrhythmias

## MYOCARDIAL INFARCTION

Transmural MI

- Entire thickness of the myocardium is destroyed (endocardium to epicardium)
- Often called Q-wave (producing) infarction as it usually produces, or is associated with changes in, the Q wave on the ECG

Subendocardial MI

- Subendocardial layer involved, does not extend through to the epicardial wall (only the inner layer of the ventricle involved)
- Often called non-Q-wave (producing) infarction

## MYOCARDIAL INFARCTION

Signs and symptoms of pulmonary congestion include:

- dyspnea
- cyanosis
- tachypnea
- frothy sputum
- labored respirations
- jugular venous distention

## MYOCARDIAL INFARCTION

Relief of pain:

- decreases anxiety and pain
- decreases myocardial oxygen demand
- decreases the risk of cardiac dysrhythmias
- may decrease heart rate and blood pressure

## MYOCARDIAL INFARCTION

Myocardial infarction is defined as necrosis (death) of some mass of the heart muscle due to an inadequate blood supply.

## MYOCARDIAL INFARCTION

- Hypertension may increase myocardial oxygen demand.
- Hypertension may exacerbate myocardial ischemia or infarction.

## MYOCARDIAL INFARCTION

- <70 years of age
- ST-segment elevation equal to or greater than 1 mm (0.1 mV) in two or more contiguous leads (II, III, aVF; I and aVL; V1 to V6).
- History of new-onset chest pain unrelieved by sublingual nitroglycerin lasting at least 30 minutes
- Seen within 6 hours of symptom onset
- No absolute contraindications to thrombolytic therapy.

## MYOCARDIAL INFARCTION

What is the significance of the American Heart Association's classification of therapeutic interventions?

## MYOCARDIAL INFARCTION

Name three goals of thrombolytic therapy.

## MYOCARDIAL INFARCTION

Name the four components of the Chain of Survival.

## MYOCARDIAL INFARCTION

- A 72 year old male is complaining of severe chest pain and weakness that has been present for approximately 3 hours. On a 1-10 scale, he rates his pain a 10.
- He is pale, and profusely diaphoretic. The skin is cool to the touch. His blood pressure is 62/40. The cardiac monitor reveals a sinus rhythm at 90 beats per minute without ectopy. Breath sounds are clear bilaterally.
- He has no significant past medical history and takes no medications regularly.
- How will you manage this patient?

## MYOCARDIAL INFARCTION

The greatest risk of death from heart attack occurs within __ after symptom onset.

## MYOCARDIAL INFARCTION

Name four modifiable risk factors.

## MYOCARDIAL INFARCTION

Name four non-modifiable risk factors.

## MYOCARDIAL INFARCTION

What are the components of Advanced Cardiac Life Support (ACLS)?

## MYOCARDIAL INFARCTION

The goals of thrombolytic therapy include:
- decreasing mortality
- improving myocardial oxygenation
- limiting the zones of myocardial ischemia
- improving perfusion to the infarct-related artery
- improving left ventricular function and cardiac output
- reducing the incidence of dysrhythmias associated with myocardial ischemia.

## MYOCARDIAL INFARCTION

Where possible, the American Heart Association's recommendations are based on the strength of supporting scientific evidence.
- Class I - definitely helpful
- Class IIa - probably helpful
- Class IIb - possibly helpful
- Class III - not indicated, may be harmful

## MYOCARDIAL INFARCTION

- This patient is most likely experiencing an acute MI and is exhibiting signs and symptoms of cardiogenic shock.
- Administer oxygen and establish IV access. Since there are no signs of pulmonary edema, administer a fluid challenge of 250 ml of normal saline. If the response is inadequate, administer a norepinephrine infusion and titrate until the systolic BP is 70-100 mm Hg.
- Once the systolic BP has increased to 70-100 mm Hg, attempt to switch to an infusion of dopamine (2.5-20 mcg/kg/min).

## MYOCARDIAL INFARCTION

- Early Access
- Early CPR
- Early Defibrillation
- Early ACLS

## MYOCARDIAL INFARCTION

Modifiable risk factors include:
- stress
- obesity
- diabetes
- hypertension
- lack of exercise
- cigarette smoking
- elevated cholesterol levels
- elevated triglyceride levels

## MYOCARDIAL INFARCTION

The greatest risk of death from heart attack occurs within the first two hours after onset of symptoms.

## MYOCARDIAL INFARCTION

The components of ACLS include Basic Life Support and:
- cardiac monitoring
- administration of drugs
- establishment of IV access
- adjunctive equipment in supporting ventilation
- defibrillation or other control of dysrhythmias
- care after resuscitation
- establishment of communication necessary to ensure continued care.

## MYOCARDIAL INFARCTION

Non-modifiable risk factors include:
- age
- race
- heredity
- male gender

## MYOCARDIAL INFARCTION

Define "afterload."

## MYOCARDIAL INFARCTION

What is meant by the term "pulseless electrical activity?"

## MYOCARDIAL INFARCTION

Why is tachycardia often associated with right-sided heart failure?

## MYOCARDIAL INFARCTION

A 70 year old male has suffered a cardiac arrest. The cardiac monitor displays ventricular tachycardia. Examination confirms the patient is pulseless and apneic.

Name four medications that may be employed in the management of this patient.

## MYOCARDIAL INFARCTION

Why is nitroglycerin administered to patients with acute pulmonary edema who have a systolic blood pressure > 100 mm Hg?

## MYOCARDIAL INFARCTION

Describe the characteristics of unstable angina.

## MYOCARDIAL INFARCTION

Which chamber of the heart is most often involved in acute myocardial infarction?

## MYOCARDIAL INFARCTION

Name two medications that may be useful in the management of acute myocardial infarction associated with hypertension.

## MYOCARDIAL INFARCTION

Pulseless electrical activity occurs when an organized rhythm with an adequate rate is seen on the cardiac monitor but no detectable pulse is produced.

## MYOCARDIAL INFARCTION

Afterload is the force or resistance against which the heart must pump to eject blood.

## MYOCARDIAL INFARCTION

Medications that may be administered in the management of pulseless VT are:

- Epinephrine
- Lidocaine
- Bretylium
- Magnesium sulfate
- Procainamide
- Sodium bicarbonate
  - If known preexisting hyperkalemia (Class I)

## MYOCARDIAL INFARCTION

The body attempts to maintain cardiac output by increasing heart rate.

The increased heart rate, however, results in decreased ventricular filling time.

## MYOCARDIAL INFARCTION

Unstable angina (also called preinfarction angina, crescendo angina) is characterized by one or more of the following:

- angina at rest or during minimal exercise
- angina of new onset, precipitated by minimal exertion
- a progressive increase in the frequency, severity and/or duration of anginal attacks in a patient with a previously stable pattern of anginal pain.

## MYOCARDIAL INFARCTION

Nitroglycerin is administered to the patient with acute pulmonary edema (with a systolic BP > 100) to increase venous capacitance (promote venous pooling), thereby reducing preload (the amount of blood returning to the right atrium) and afterload (the resistance against which the heart must pump to eject blood).

## MYOCARDIAL INFARCTION

- Relief of pain and anxiety with morphine or sublingual nitroglycerin.
- If pulmonary congestion is present, furosemide.
- If unresponsive to initial therapy, consider IV nitroglycerin (esp. if CHF is present) or beta-blockers in tachycardia and high cardiac output.
- IV nitroprusside may be considered when ischemia is absent.

## MYOCARDIAL INFARCTION

The left ventricle is the chamber of the heart most often involved in acute myocardial infarction.

## MYOCARDIAL INFARCTION

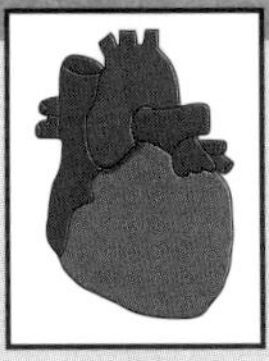

Describe effects of parasympathetic stimulation of the heart.

## MYOCARDIAL INFARCTION

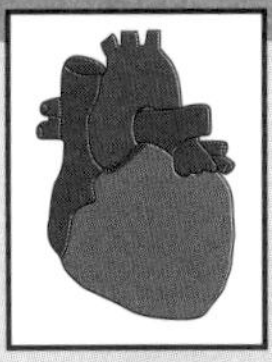

Patients who experience a(n) _____ myocardial infarction have a greater incidence of congestive heart failure and cardiogenic shock than those who have MIs affecting other areas of the left ventricle.

## MYOCARDIAL INFARCTION

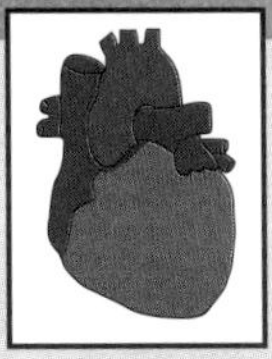

Tachycardia, jugular venous distention, dyspnea, diaphoresis and dependent edema are signs and symptoms of _____ heart failure.

## MYOCARDIAL INFARCTION

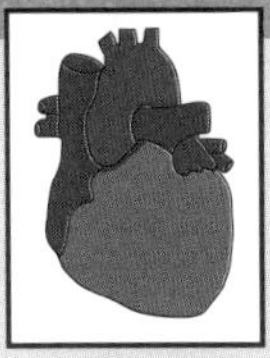

Name three signs and symptoms of cardiogenic shock.

## MYOCARDIAL INFARCTION

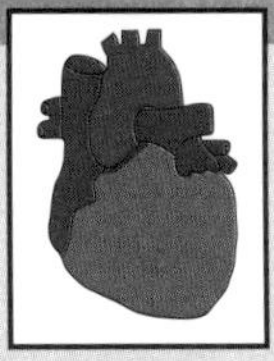

Name three causes of cardiac arrest other than atherosclerotic heart disease.

## MYOCARDIAL INFARCTION

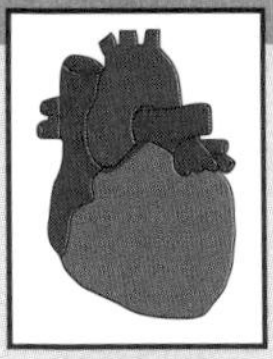

What is Prinzmetal's angina?

## MYOCARDIAL INFARCTION

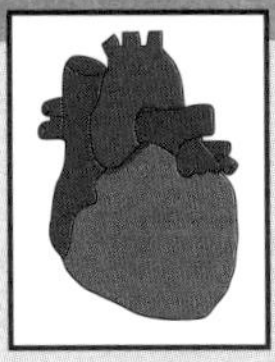

As the right ventricle contracts, Blood is pumped through the _____ valve to the _____ artery.

## MYOCARDIAL INFARCTION

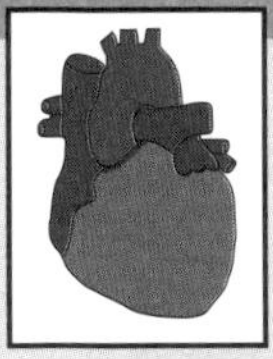

Anterior or lateral wall infarctions are most often due to occlusion of the __ coronary artery.

## MYOCARDIAL INFARCTION

- Patients who experience an anterior MI have a greater incidence of congestive heart failure and cardiogenic shock than those who have MIs affecting other areas of the left ventricle.
- Anterior MI is also associated with a higher mortality rate.

## MYOCARDIAL INFARCTION

Stimulation of parasympathetic nerve fibers causes the release of acetylcholine which results in:
- a slowing of the rate of discharge of the sinus node
- a decrease in the rate of conduction through the AV node
- resulting in a decrease in heart rate.

## MYOCARDIAL INFARCTION

- Hypotension
- Cool, clammy skin
- Signs and symptoms of acute MI.
- Sinus tachycardia is the most common rhythm seen.
- Altered level of consciousness which may include restlessness, confusion or unconsciousness.

## MYOCARDIAL INFARCTION

- These are signs and symptoms of right heart failure.
- Other signs and symptoms of right heart failure include:
  - Dyspnea
  - Diaphoresis
  - Tachycardia
  - Dependent edema
  - Jugular venous distention
- Fatigue (due to decreased cardiac output)

## MYOCARDIAL INFARCTION

- Prinzmetal's angina (also known as variant angina, resting angina) is a spontaneous type of anginal pain that is thought to be due to coronary artery spasm typically associated with marked ST segment elevation on the ECG.
- Commonly occurs at rest between the hours of midnight and 8 a.m.
- Usually relieved with nitroglycerin.
- May be accompanied by acute MI.

## MYOCARDIAL INFARCTION

- Trauma
- Hypoxia
- Drowning
- Electrocution
- Hypothermia
- Drug overdose
- Acid-base imbalance
- Electrolyte imbalance

## MYOCARDIAL INFARCTION

Anterior or lateral wall infarctions are most often due to occlusion of the left coronary artery.

## MYOCARDIAL INFARCTION

As the right ventricle contracts, blood is pumped through the pulmonary semilunar valve to the pulmonary artery.

## MYOCARDIAL INFARCTION

- A 65 year old female is complaining of difficulty breathing. She is awake, extremely anxious and laboring to breathe. Examination reveals a BP of 166/94, irregular pulse rate of 90-120 beats/minute and a respiratory rate of 32. The skin is cool and moist. Auscultation of the chest reveals bilateral crackles and pitting edema of the ankles is noted. The cardiac monitor shows atrial fibrillation. The patient has a history of hypertension for which she takes Catapres.
- How will you manage this patient?

## MYOCARDIAL INFARCTION

What is the key question that should be asked for every patient with shock or hypotension?

## MYOCARDIAL INFARCTION

What are the components of the "cardiovascular triad?"

## MYOCARDIAL INFARCTION

An 83 year old female in acute pulmonary edema has a blood pressure of 78/44. The cardiac monitor shows a sinus tachycardia at 110 beats/minute.

Describe your management of this patient.

## MYOCARDIAL INFARCTION

A 56 year old male has suffered a myocardial infarction in which the full thickness of the heart wall was involved.

What is the name given to this type of myocardial infarction?

## MYOCARDIAL INFARCTION

What is the most common complication in the first few hours of acute myocardial infarction?

## MYOCARDIAL INFARCTION

Name three second-line medications used in the treatment of acute pulmonary edema.

## MYOCARDIAL INFARCTION

Hypotension may occur during acute myocardial infarction for several reasons.

Name four possible causes of hypotension associated with a rate problem.

## MYOCARDIAL INFARCTION

For every patient with shock or hypotension, one should ask, "Is there a rate problem, a pump problem, or a volume problem?"

Emergency Cardiac Care Committee and Subcommittees, American Heart Association. Guidelines for cardiopulmonary resuscitation and emergency cardiac care, JAMA 268:2227, 1992.

## MYOCARDIAL INFARCTION

This patient is suffering from acute pulmonary edema. First-line treatment measures should include:

- Sit the patient up with the legs dependent
- Administer oxygen (be prepared to intubate if necessary)
- Establish IV access
- Administer furosemide 0.5-1.0 mg/kg
- Administer sublingual nitroglycerin
- Consider morphine administration

## MYOCARDIAL INFARCTION

- Initiate oxygen therapy, establish IV access and prepare a dopamine infusion.
    - Dopamine is the drug of choice for hypotension with a systolic blood pressure between 70 and 100 mm Hg.
- Dopamine should be started at 2.5-5 mcg/kg/minute and titrated as needed to 20 mcg/kg/minute.

## MYOCARDIAL INFARCTION

The cardiovascular triad consists of the:

- myocardium
- vascular system
- conducting system

## MYOCARDIAL INFARCTION

The most common complication in the first few hours of acute myocardial infarction is cardiac dysrhythmias, thus the reason ECG monitoring is essential.

## MYOCARDIAL INFARCTION

A myocardial infarction involving the full thickness of the myocardium is called a transmural infarction.

- This type of infarction may also be called a Q-wave (producing) infarction as it usually produces, or is associated with changes in, the Q wave on the ECG.

## MYOCARDIAL INFARCTION

- Rate too fast:
    - Sinus tachycardia
    - Atrial fibrillation
    - Atrial flutter
    - PSVT
    - Ventricular tachycardia
- Rate too slow:
    - Sinus bradycardia
    - Second-degree AV block, type I
    - Second-degree AV block, type II
    - Third-degree AV block
    - Pacemaker failure

## MYOCARDIAL INFARCTION

Second-line medications used in the treatment of acute pulmonary edema include:

- IV nitroglycerin (if systolic BP > 100)
- Nitroprusside (if systolic BP > 100)
- Dopamine (if systolic BP < 100)
- Dobutamine (if normotensive)

## MYOCARDIAL INFARCTION

Name the most common rhythm seen in the first minute of out-of-hospital adult cardiac arrest.

## MYOCARDIAL INFARCTION

Cardiogenic shock is most often due to extensive myocardial infarction, involving approximately __% or more of the left ventricle.

## MYOCARDIAL INFARCTION

- A 60 year old male is complaining of severe chest pain present for the past 40 minutes unrelieved with rest. He describes his pain as a sensation like a "rubber band wrapped around my chest."
- His blood pressure is 66/40 and the cardiac monitor shows a sinus bradycardia with occasional uniform PVCs.
- How will you manage this patient?

## MYOCARDIAL INFARCTION

Name the three primary goals of management of myocardial infarction.

## MYOCARDIAL INFARCTION

Inferior wall myocardial infarction is usually the result of occlusion of the ____ coronary artery.

## MYOCARDIAL INFARCTION

Name four signs and symptoms of pulmonary edema.

## MYOCARDIAL INFARCTION

Name two signs of pericardial tamponade.

## MYOCARDIAL INFARCTION

A 77 year old female has suffered a cardiac arrest. When performing a quick-look, you are unsure if the rhythm shown on the cardiac monitor is asystole or fine ventricular fibrillation.

How should you proceed?

## MYOCARDIAL INFARCTION

Cardiogenic shock is most often due to extensive myocardial infarction, involving approximately 40% or more of the left ventricle.

## MYOCARDIAL INFARCTION

The most common rhythm seen in the first minute of out-of-hospital adult cardiac arrest is ventricular fibrillation.

## MYOCARDIAL INFARCTION

The three primary goals of management of acute myocardial infarction are:

- relief of pain and anxiety
- limitation of infarct size
- prevention of life-threatening dysrhythmias.

## MYOCARDIAL INFARCTION

- Administer oxygen and establish IV access.
- Administer atropine 0.5-1.0 mg rapid IV bolus and reassess.
- Medication for relief of pain should be withheld until the patient's systolic blood pressure is 100 mm Hg or greater.

## MYOCARDIAL INFARCTION

Signs and symptoms of acute pulmonary edema include:

- tachycardia
- diaphoresis
- pink, foamy sputum
- severe respiratory distress
- severe agitation/confusion
- rales, rhonchi, possible wheezes
- hyper- or hypotension may be present
- chest pain may or may not be present

## MYOCARDIAL INFARCTION

Inferior wall myocardial infarction is usually the result of occlusion of the right coronary artery.

## MYOCARDIAL INFARCTION

If you are unsure if the rhythm is asystole or fine ventricular fibrillation, treat as if the rhythm is VF and defibrillate.

## MYOCARDIAL INFARCTION

Signs of pericardial tamponade include:

- hypotension
- pulsus paradoxus
- distended neck veins
- muffled heart sounds
- narrowing pulse pressure

## MYOCARDIAL INFARCTION

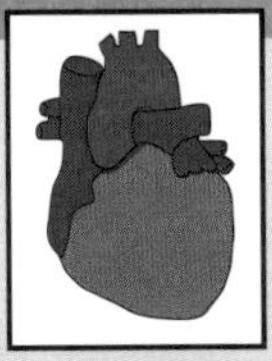

High levels of creatine kinase are common following resuscitation. What is the reason for this?

## MYOCARDIAL INFARCTION

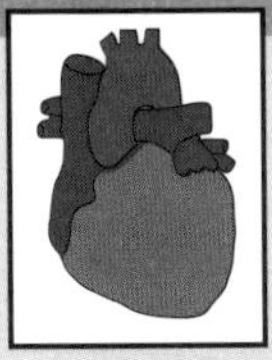

Metabolic causes should be considered as a possible precipitating cause of cardiac arrest if postresuscitation serial ECGs fail to demonstrate evidence for acute infarction.

Name two possible metabolic causes of cardiac arrest.

## MYOCARDIAL INFARCTION

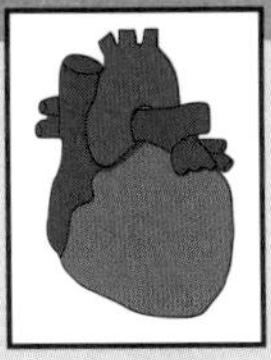

- Thrombolysis occurs approximately 30-45 minutes after initiation of thrombolytic therapy.
- Although proof of coronary artery reperfusion requires coronary angiography, this is not always possible or practical.
- Name two practical clinical indicators of reperfusion.

## MYOCARDIAL INFARCTION

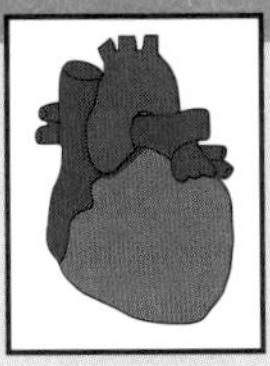

Describe the ECG changes seen in acute myocardial infarction.

## MYOCARDIAL INFARCTION

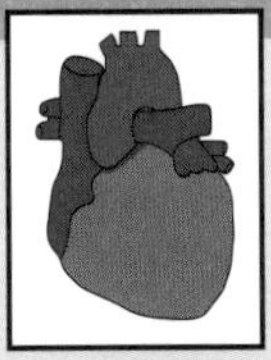

What types of dysrhythmias are particularly common with an inferior wall MI?

## MYOCARDIAL INFARCTION

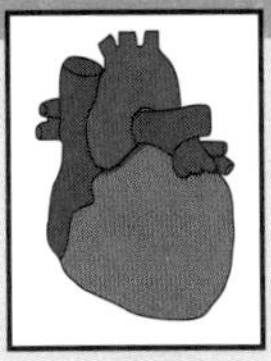

Name three complications of myocardial infarction.

## MYOCARDIAL INFARCTION

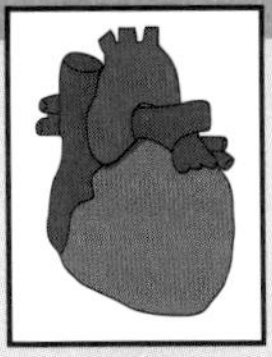

Describe the effects of cocaine on the cardiovascular system.

## MYOCARDIAL INFARCTION

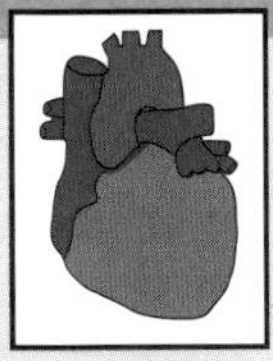

After initiating thrombolytic therapy, the patient should be observed for signs suggestive of reperfusion.

What is meant by the term "reperfusion dysrhythmias"?

## MYOCARDIAL INFARCTION

Inferior wall MIs are frequently associated with:
- sinus bradycardia
- first-degree AV block
- second-degree AV block, type I (Wenckebach)
- complete (third-degree) AV block with a junctional escape rhythm

## MYOCARDIAL INFARCTION

The creatine kinase elevation is presumably due to skeletal muscle trauma secondary to chest compression during CPR and to cardiac muscle ischemia during arrest and attempted resuscitation.

## MYOCARDIAL INFARCTION

- Dysrhythmias (most common)
- Pericarditis
- Thromboembolism
- Cardiogenic shock
- Congestive heart failure
- Muscle dysfunction
  - ventricular wall rupture
  - ventricular aneurysm
  - papillary muscle rupture or dysfunction

## MYOCARDIAL INFARCTION

- The most common include:
  - recent initiation of antidysrhythmic drug treatment
  - hypokalemia
- Other possible metabolic abnormalities include:
  - hypothermia
  - hypomagnesemia
  - toxic reactions to phenothiazines, cocaine and cyclic antidepressants.

## MYOCARDIAL INFARCTION

- Cocaine use results in sympathomimetic effects such as:
  - increased heart rate
  - increased myocardial contractility
  - increased blood pressure.
- These effects may result in:
  - hypertension
  - myocardial infarction
  - cardiac dysrhythmias
  - precipitation of angina
  - coronary artery vasospasm.

## MYOCARDIAL INFARCTION

- Relief of chest pain or ischemic symptoms
  - Relief is often abrupt, occurring 30-90 minutes after initiation of thrombolytic therapy.
- Normalization of ST segments.
  - An indicator of acute MI is ST segment elevation of 1 mm or more in two contiguous leads.
  - Normalization of the ST segment may take up to 24 hours to occur after thrombolytic therapy.
- Reperfusion dysrhythmias
  - Most common are VT, sinus bradycardia and accelerated idioventricular rhythm.

## MYOCARDIAL INFARCTION

- Reperfusion refers to the return of oxygenated blood to ischemic myocardial tissue.
- "Reperfusion dysrhythmias" refers to abnormal rhythms seen once blood flow is reestablished to ischemic heart muscle.

## MYOCARDIAL INFARCTION

- The zone of ischemia produces symmetrical T-wave inversion due to altered tissue repolarization.
- The zone of injury produces ST segment elevation due to abnormal repolarization.
- The zone of infarction (necrosis) produces abnormal Q waves due to the lack of depolarization of necrotic tissue.

## MYOCARDIAL INFARCTION

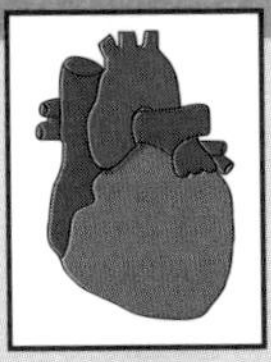

Describe the pain pattern typically associated with chronic stable angina.

## MYOCARDIAL INFARCTION

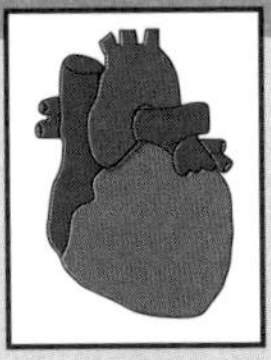

Explain why the use of calcium channel blockers may be beneficial in the management of angina or acute myocardial infarction.

## MYOCARDIAL INFARCTION

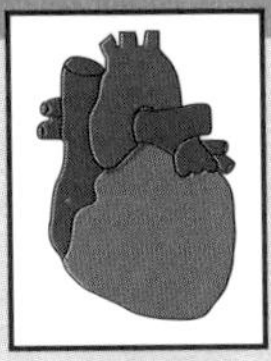

Name the main branches of:

- the right coronary artery
- the left coronary artery.

## MYOCARDIAL INFARCTION

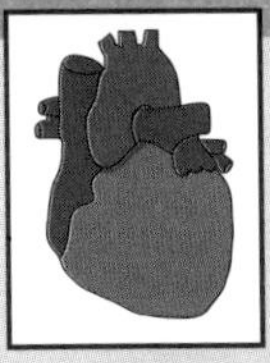

- A 63 year old female is complaining of chest pain and a severe headache. Her blood pressure is 240/146, pulse 110, respirations 18-20. Nifedipine, 10 mg, is ordered for administration to this patient.
- What type of drug is Nifedipine?
- Explain how this medication may be beneficial in the management of this patient.

## MYOCARDIAL INFARCTION

Calcium channel blockers:

- cause dilation of the coronary arteries
    - resulting in increased blood flow.
- relax vascular smooth muscle resulting in vasodilation
    - vasodilation results in a decrease in afterload (the resistance against which the heart must pump).
- decrease myocardial oxygen demand.

## MYOCARDIAL INFARCTION

- The pain associated with chronic stable angina is predictable and consistent.
- Precipitating factors include exertion/exercise, cold weather, emotional stress.
- Pain is usually relieved with rest or within 45 seconds to 5 minutes of nitroglycerin administration.

## MYOCARDIAL INFARCTION

- Nifedipine (Procardia, Adalat) is a calcium channel blocker used in the management of hypertensive emergencies and in patients with ischemic chest pain who remain symptomatic despite nitroglycerin therapy or who cannot tolerate nitroglycerin.
- Nifedipine causes vasodilation of the peripheral vasculature and coronary arteries resulting in a decrease in afterload.
- Nifedipine is usually administered by puncturing the capsule with a sterile needle and squeezing the contents under the patient's tongue. The patient may also bite the capsule and swallow it to enhance absorption of the drug.

## MYOCARDIAL INFARCTION

- The main branches of the right coronary artery are the:
    - marginal artery
    - posterior descending artery
- The main branches of the left coronary artery are the:
    - circumflex artery
    - anterior descending artery.

## AIRWAY MANAGEMENT

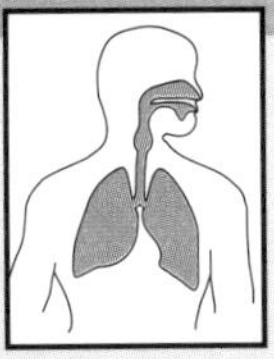

Name four possible complications of surgical cricothyroidotomy.

## AIRWAY MANAGEMENT

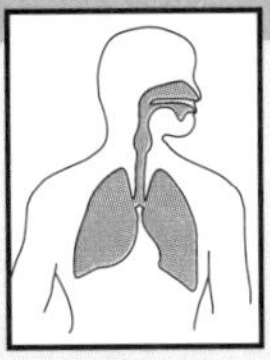

Name two advantages of the pharyngotracheal lumen airway (PtLA).

## AIRWAY MANAGEMENT

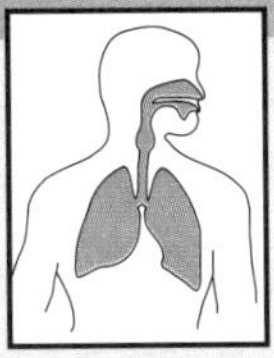

Name five desirable features of a bag-valve-mask device.

## AIRWAY MANAGEMENT

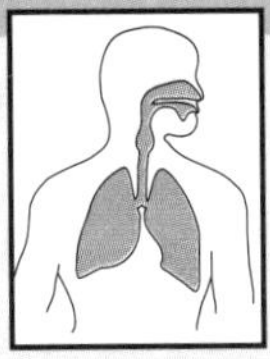

An endotracheal intubation attempt should not take more than 30 seconds.

At what point does this 30 second time interval begin and end?

## AIRWAY MANAGEMENT

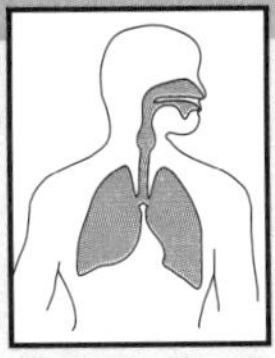

Name two advantages of pulse oximetry.

## AIRWAY MANAGEMENT

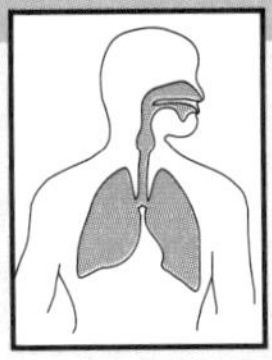

State the equipment needed for insertion of the esophageal obturator airway (EOA).

## AIRWAY MANAGEMENT

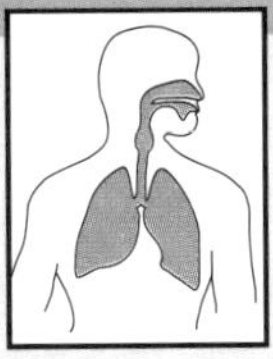

What is the purpose of cricoid pressure (the Sellick maneuver)?

## AIRWAY MANAGEMENT

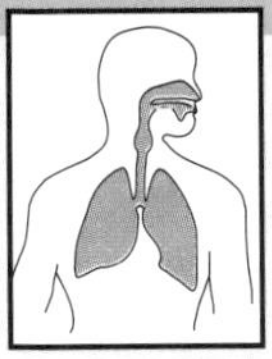

Name five possible complications of endotracheal intubation.

## AIRWAY MANAGEMENT

- Visualization of the airway is not required for insertion.
- Because of the oropharyngeal balloon, the need for a face mask is eliminated.
- Reasonable technique to use in suspected neck injury since the head does not have to be hyperextended.

## AIRWAY MANAGEMENT

- Asphyxia
- Hoarseness
- Aspiration of blood
- Vocal cord paralysis
- Mediastinal emphysema
- Hemorrhage or hematoma formation
- Laceration of the trachea/esophagus
- Creation of a false passage into the tissues

## AIRWAY MANAGEMENT

The 30 second time interval begins when ventilation of the patient ceases to allow insertion of the laryngoscope blade into the patient's mouth and ends when the patient is reventilated upon placement of the endotracheal tube.

## AIRWAY MANAGEMENT

- A clear mask
- NO pop-off valve
- A true nonrebreathing valve
- Available in both adult and pediatric sizes
- Self-inflating bag that is easily cleaned and sterilized
- Must perform satisfactorily under all common environmental conditions and extremes of temperature
- A system for delivering high concentrations of oxygen through an oxygen reservoir or oxygen inlet at the back of the bag

## AIRWAY MANAGEMENT

- Gloves, mask, protective eye wear
- Esophageal obturator airway (or esophageal gastric tube airway)
- 35 ml syringe
- Suction device
- Stethoscope
- Water-soluble lubricant
- Bag-valve device with reservoir and oxygen source.

## AIRWAY MANAGEMENT

- Painless
- Noninvasive
- Does not require drawing or handling of blood
- Can provide a continuous measurement of oxygenation.

## AIRWAY MANAGEMENT

- Cuff leak
- Aspiration
- Dysrhythmias
- Laryngospasm
- Bronchospasm
- Inadvertent esophageal intubation
- Obstruction of the endotracheal tube
- Inadvertent right mainstem bronchus intubation
- Hypoxia due to prolonged or unsuccessful intubation
- Trauma to the lips, teeth, tongue or soft tissues of the oropharynx.

## AIRWAY MANAGEMENT

Cricoid pressure (the Sellick maneuver) may be applied to:

- minimize gastric distention and aspiration
- aid placement of an endotracheal tube into the tracheal opening.

## AIRWAY MANAGEMENT

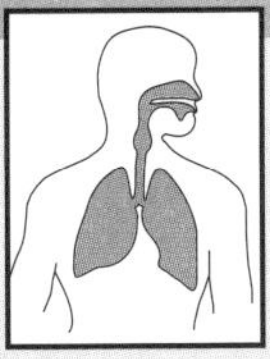

What is a stylet and what is its purpose?

## AIRWAY MANAGEMENT

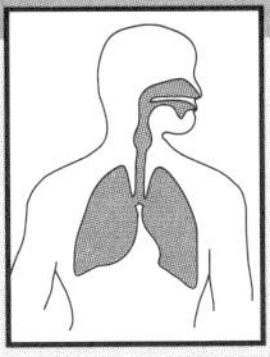

Name four advantages of endotracheal intubation.

## AIRWAY MANAGEMENT

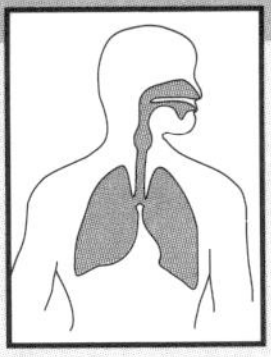

What is the average endotracheal tube size for:

- an adult male?
- an adult female?

## AIRWAY MANAGEMENT

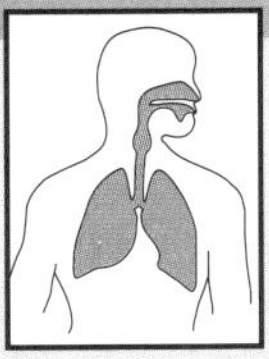

A 64 year old male in respiratory failure has just been intubated.

How will you confirm correct placement of the endotracheal tube?

## AIRWAY MANAGEMENT

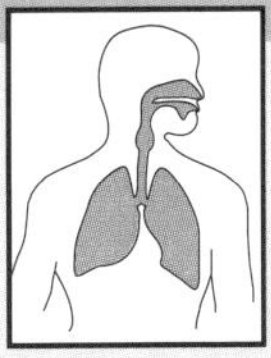

When are chest thrusts recommended in the treatment of a foreign body airway obstruction?

## AIRWAY MANAGEMENT

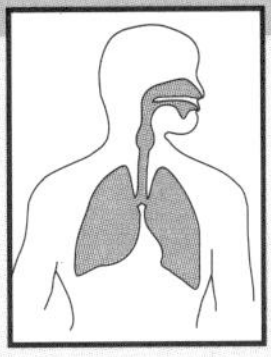

An advantage of ventilation with a bag-valve device is a sense of compliance of the lungs is conveyed to the operator.

What is meant by the term "compliance"?

## AIRWAY MANAGEMENT

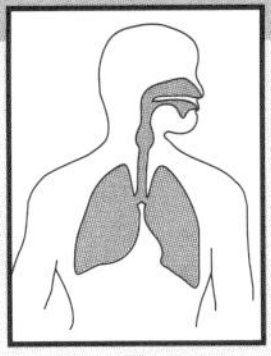

Name the disadvantages associated with the use of the pharyngotracheal lumen airway (PtLA).

## AIRWAY MANAGEMENT

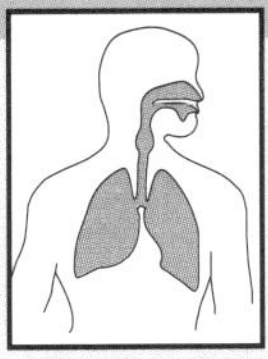

Describe two methods for insertion of an oropharyngeal airway (OPA) in an adult.

## AIRWAY MANAGEMENT

Chest thrusts are recommended in the treatment of a foreign body airway obstruction if the victim is markedly obese or in cases of advanced pregnancy.

## AIRWAY MANAGEMENT

- A stylet is a plastic-coated metal wire that may be inserted inside an endotracheal tube prior to an endotracheal intubation attempt.
- The stylet allows the endotracheal tube to be shaped to any desired configuration.
  - The tip of the stylet must be recessed at least 1/2 inch from the end of the endotracheal tube to avoid trauma to the anatomical structures of the airway.

## AIRWAY MANAGEMENT

- Compliance refers to the resistance of the patient's lung tissue to ventilation.
- For example, lung compliance is reduced in tension pneumothorax resulting in increased resistance (poor compliance) = harder to ventilate the patient.

## AIRWAY MANAGEMENT

- Isolates the airway
- Keeps the airway patent
- Reduces the risk of aspiration
- Permits suctioning of the trachea
- Ensures delivery of a high concentration of oxygen
- Provides a route for administration of some medications
- Ensures delivery of an adequate tidal volume to maintain lung inflation.

## AIRWAY MANAGEMENT

- Reports of an inadequate seal with the pharyngeal balloon.
- Design of the device may pose a problem when attempting to replace the PtLA with a tracheal tube.

## AIRWAY MANAGEMENT

The average endotracheal tube size for an adult male is 8-8.5 internal diameter (i.d.) and 7.5-8.0 for an adult female.

## AIRWAY MANAGEMENT

- The OPA is inserted upside down (with the tip pointing toward the roof of the mouth) into the mouth. When the distal end reaches the soft palate, the airway is rotated 180 degrees and slipped behind the tongue into the posterior pharynx.
- A tongue blade may be used to depress the tongue. If this method is used, the OPA is inserted right side up into the oropharynx.

## AIRWAY MANAGEMENT

- Observe the rise and fall of the chest.
- Perform a five-point auscultation:
  - Auscultate breath sounds of the left and right lung fields at the apices and the anterior bases.
  - Auscultate the epigastrium (should be silent).

## AIRWAY MANAGEMENT

A nasal cannula (prongs) with a liter flow of 1-6 liters/minute will deliver what percentage of oxygen?

## AIRWAY MANAGEMENT

You are attempting to intubate an adult patient who has suffered a respiratory arrest. A capable assistant is applying cricoid pressure.

At what point should cricoid pressure be released?

## AIRWAY MANAGEMENT

Describe the technique for performing a jaw thrust.

## AIRWAY MANAGEMENT

What is the carina?

## AIRWAY MANAGEMENT

Name three signs of poor air exchange associated with a partial airway obstruction.

## AIRWAY MANAGEMENT

Describe the recommended sequence of events to be employed when treating the conscious adult (standing) with a suspected complete airway obstruction.

## AIRWAY MANAGEMENT

Name three advantages of automatic transport ventilators (ATVs).

## AIRWAY MANAGEMENT

What is the minimum oxygen flow rate that should be used with a simple face mask?

## AIRWAY MANAGEMENT

Cricoid pressure should be maintained until the cuff of the endotracheal tube is inflated.

## AIRWAY MANAGEMENT

- A nasal cannula can deliver an oxygen concentration of 25-45% at a flow rate of 1-6 liters/minute.
- The formula to calculate the O2 percentage at a given liter flow is 21% (room air) + 4 x oxygen flow in liters/minute
  - 1 liter/minute = 25%
  - 2 liters/minute = 29%
  - 3 liters/minute = 33%
  - 4 liters/minute = 37%
  - 5 liters/minute = 41%
  - 6 liters/minute = 45%

## AIRWAY MANAGEMENT

The carina is the point where the trachea bifurcates into the right and left mainstem bronchi.

- approximately the level of the sternal angle (angle of Louis) anteriorly
- approximately the level of the 5th or 6th thoracic vertebrae posteriorly

## AIRWAY MANAGEMENT

- The rescuer's index fingers are bent and placed at the angles of the patient's jaw.
- When the jaw is lifted upward, the chin is moved forward and the tongue displaced away from the posterior pharynx.

## AIRWAY MANAGEMENT

- Ask, Are you choking?
- Assure the victim you are going to assist him/her
- Stand behind the victim and perform abdominal thrusts
  - Wrap your arms around the victim's waist
  - Make a fist with one hand (thumbside placed against the victim's abdomen in the midline slightly above the navel and well below the tip of the xiphoid)
  - Grasp the fist with your other hand and deliver quick, upward thrusts
- Continue until the object is expelled or the victim loses consciousness.

## AIRWAY MANAGEMENT

Signs of poor air exchange associated with a partial airway obstruction include:

- possible cyanosis
- weak, ineffective cough
- increased respiratory difficulty
- high-pitched noise while inhaling

## AIRWAY MANAGEMENT

When using a simple face mask, the oxygen flow rate must be higher than 5 liters per minute to avoid the accumulation of exhaled air in the mask reservoir that might be rebreathed.

## AIRWAY MANAGEMENT

- Free the rescuer for other tasks when used in intubated patients.
- Cricoid pressure can be applied with one hand while the other seals the mask on the face.
- Once set, can provide a specific tidal volume, respiratory rate and minute ventilation.
- Improved lung inflation with diminished or absent gastric insufflation due to lower inspiratory flow rates and longer inspiratory times provided by the device.

## AIRWAY MANAGEMENT

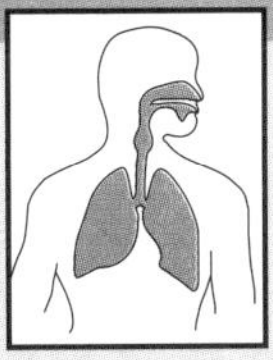

A 78 year old female has suffered a respiratory arrest. You have intubated the patient and note there is an absence of chest wall movement with bag-valve device ventilation and you are unable to auscultate breath sounds on either side of the chest.

- What is the most likely cause of this situation?
- What corrective action will you initiate?

## AIRWAY MANAGEMENT

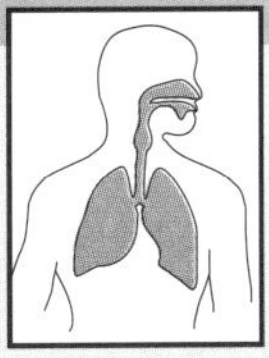

- What is tidal volume?
- How is it assessed?

## AIRWAY MANAGEMENT

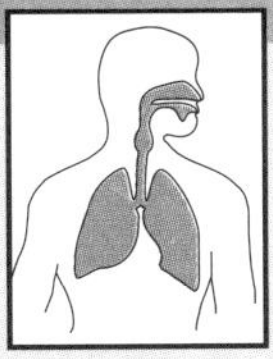

What is the maximum length of time a patient should be suctioned at one time?

## AIRWAY MANAGEMENT

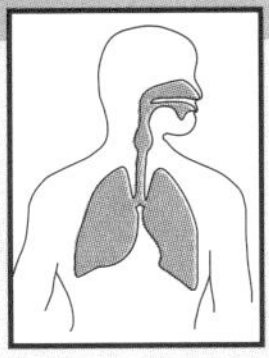

Name two advantages of ventilation with the bag-valve device.

## AIRWAY MANAGEMENT

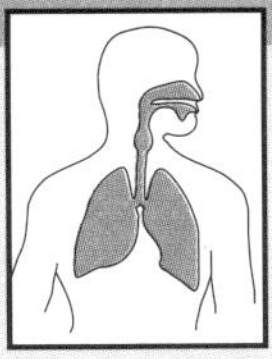

What is the maximum length of time ventilation should be interrupted for an intubation attempt?

## AIRWAY MANAGEMENT

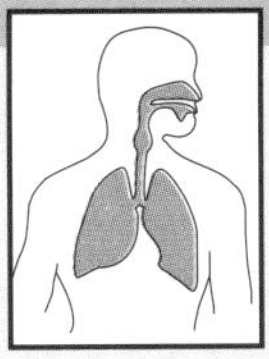

You are asked to perform a surgical cricothyroidotomy on a 50 year old patient with an airway obstruction unrelieved by other methods.

Name the landmarks you must locate in order to properly perform this procedure.

## AIRWAY MANAGEMENT

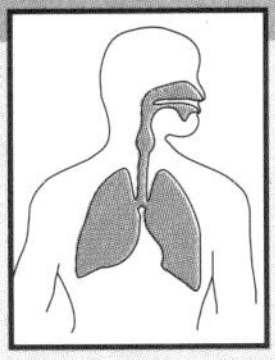

A 61 year old male has suffered a respiratory arrest. An endotracheal tube has been correctly placed and you are preparing to ventilate the patient with a bag-valve device.

What oxygen liter flow should be used when ventilating the patient with the device?

## AIRWAY MANAGEMENT

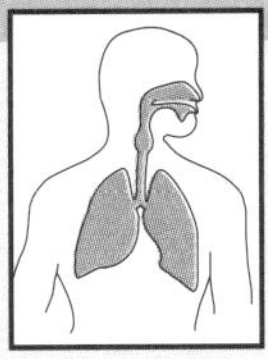

During a cardiac arrest, a bag-valve-mask device should not possess a pop-off (pressure-release) valve.

What is the reason for this?

## AIRWAY MANAGEMENT

- Tidal volume is the volume of air exchanged in a normal breath.
- At rest, the volume of one breath is about 500 ml.
- Tidal volume is assessed by chest rise and auscultation of bilateral breath sounds.

## AIRWAY MANAGEMENT

- You have most likely intubated the esophagus.
- Deflate the endotracheal tube cuff and remove the endotracheal tube.
- Hyperventilate the patient before attempting another intubation.

## AIRWAY MANAGEMENT

- Increased oxygen delivery to the patient
- Sense of compliance of the patient's lungs is conveyed to the rescuer
- Immediate ventilation of the patient with an oxygen enriched mixture
- Can be used with the spontaneously breathing patient as well as the apneic patient.

## AIRWAY MANAGEMENT

- Limit suctioning to no more than 10 seconds.
- Hyperventilate the patient before and after suctioning.

## AIRWAY MANAGEMENT

- The superior landmark is the notch at the base of the thyroid cartilage.
- The inferior landmark is the cricoid cartilage.
- The small depression below the thyroid cartilage corresponds to the cricothyroid membrane.
    - It is at this point that an incision is made (or a needle is inserted when performing a needle cricothyroidotomy).

## AIRWAY MANAGEMENT

The maximum length of time ventilation should be interrupted for an intubation attempt is 30 seconds.

## AIRWAY MANAGEMENT

- To properly ventilate patients in cardiac arrest, much higher than usual airway pressures are often needed.
- The pressure needed to overcome the increase in airway resistance may exceed the limits of the pop-off valve thus, a pop-off valve may prevent delivery of sufficient tidal volume to properly ventilate the patient in cardiac arrest.

## AIRWAY MANAGEMENT

The patient should be ventilated with the bag-valve device (with a reservoir) connected to supplemental oxygen with at least 12 liters/minute flow.

## AIRWAY MANAGEMENT

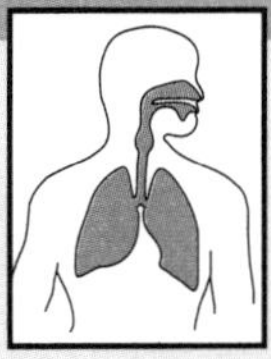

When using a pocket mask, an oxygen flow rate of 15 liters/minute will provide an inspired oxygen concentration of approximately ____%.

## AIRWAY MANAGEMENT

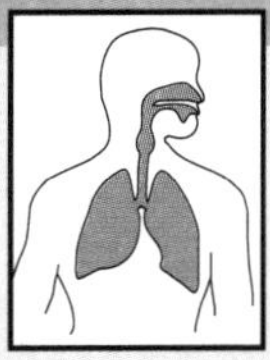

Name two possible complications of oropharyngeal airway (OPA) insertion.

## AIRWAY MANAGEMENT

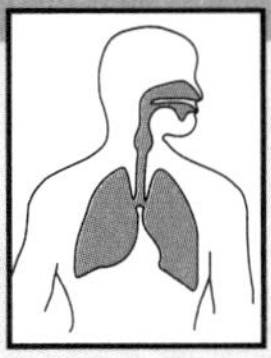

What volume of air does the cuff of the esophageal obturator hold?

## AIRWAY MANAGEMENT

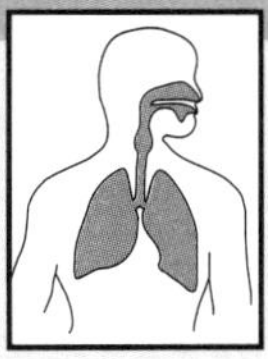

Is it necessary to maintain proper head positioning once an oropharyngeal airway (OPA) is inserted?

## AIRWAY MANAGEMENT

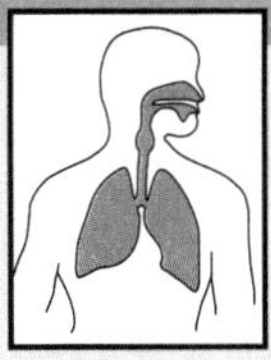

Most commercially available adult bag-valve devices are capable of storing what volume of air?

## AIRWAY MANAGEMENT

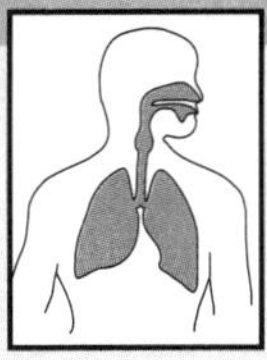

State the preferred tidal volume for ventilating the adult patient with a bag-valve device.

## AIRWAY MANAGEMENT

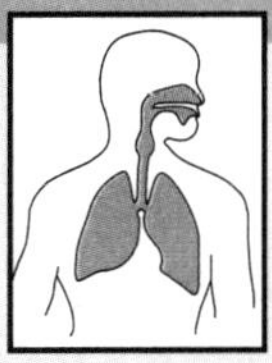

What is minute volume?

## AIRWAY MANAGEMENT

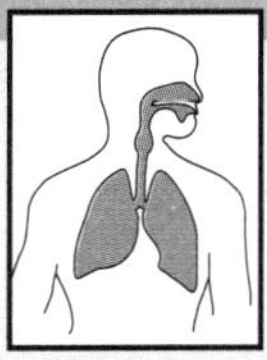

Name four signs of respiratory distress.

## AIRWAY MANAGEMENT

Possible complications of OPA insertion include:

- trauma/bleeding of the oropharynx
- bradycardia as a result of stimulation of the gag reflex
- insertion in the conscious or semiconscious patient may stimulating vomiting or laryngospasm
- if the airway is too long, it may press the epiglottis against the entrance of the larynx, producing a complete airway obstruction

## AIRWAY MANAGEMENT

When using a pocket mask, an oxygen flow rate of 15 liters/minute will provide an inspired oxygen concentration of approximately 80%.

## AIRWAY MANAGEMENT

Yes, with the oropharyngeal airway (OPA) inserted, proper head position must be maintained.

## AIRWAY MANAGEMENT

The cuff of the esophageal obturator airway (EOA) or esophageal gastric tube airway (EGTA) holds 30-35 ml of air.

## AIRWAY MANAGEMENT

A tidal volume of 10-15 ml/kg should be delivered over 2 seconds.

- Slightly more volume may be needed for the very obese patient.
- Slightly less volume may be needed for patients with fragile intrathoracic airways or diminished lung volumes.

## AIRWAY MANAGEMENT

The typical adult bag-valve device is capable of storing 1000-1600 ml of air.

- The average child bag-valve device is capable of storing 500-700 ml of air.
- The average infant bag-valve device is capable of storing 150-240 ml of air.

## AIRWAY MANAGEMENT

There are many signs of respiratory distress. Some of them are:

- nasal flaring
- tracheal tugging
- jugular venous distention
- inability to speak in full sentences
- confusion, agitation, combativeness
- dyspnea (difficult or labored breathing)
- retractions, use of accessory muscles of respiration.

## AIRWAY MANAGEMENT

Minute volume is tidal volume times the respiratory rate.

- If the minute volume is increased, the PaCO2 decreases.
  - For example, the patient with increased intracranial pressure may be hyperventilated in an attempt to blow off CO2 and promote cerebral vasoconstriction.
- If the minute volume is decreased, the PaCO2 increases.

## AIRWAY MANAGEMENT

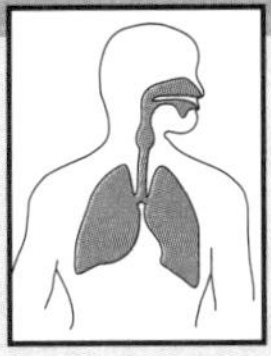

When is needle or surgical cricothyroidotomy indicated?

## AIRWAY MANAGEMENT

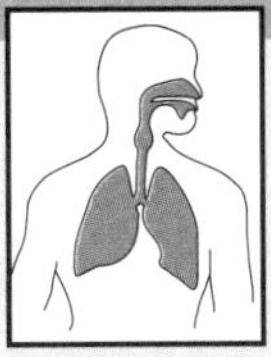

Where is the narrowest part of the airway in an adult?

## AIRWAY MANAGEMENT

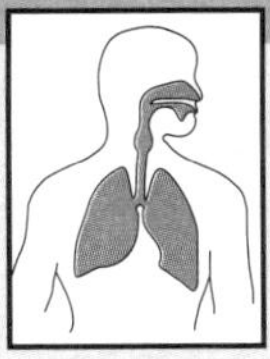

Name four contraindications for use of the esophageal obturator airway (EOA).

## AIRWAY MANAGEMENT

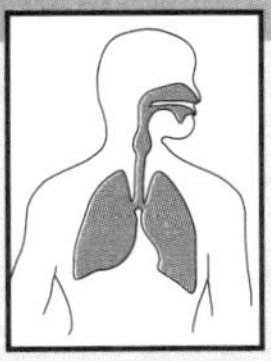

When using a pocket mask, an oxygen flow rate of 10 liters per minute will provide an inspired oxygen concentration of approximately _____%.

## AIRWAY MANAGEMENT

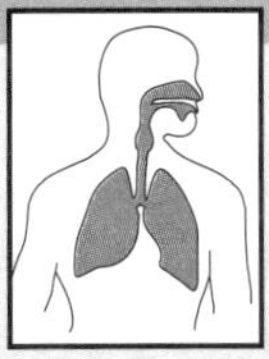

Name three possible complications of suctioning.

## AIRWAY MANAGEMENT

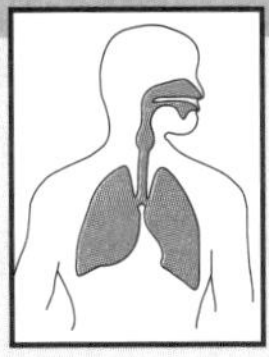

Name two disadvantages of the nasopharyngeal airway (NPA).

## AIRWAY MANAGEMENT

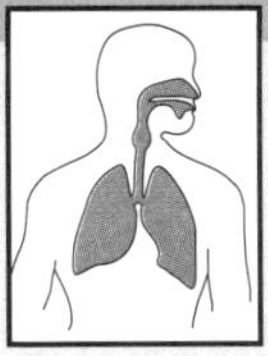

Name three indications for use of the pharyngotracheal lumen airway (PtLA).

## AIRWAY MANAGEMENT

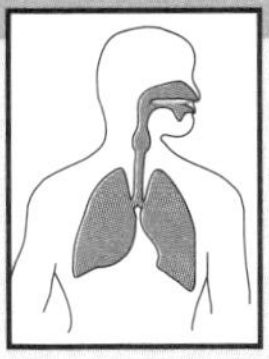

You are intubating a patient in cardiac arrest and have visualized the vocal cords.

How far should you advance the endotracheal tube beyond the vocal cords?

## AIRWAY MANAGEMENT

- Severe hypoxia
- Increased arterial pressure and tachycardia
- Bradycardia and hypotension due to vagal stimulation
- Damage to the mucosa resulting in edema, hemorrhage, ulcerated areas that may result in tracheal infection
- May trigger coughing, resulting in increased intracranial pressure and a reduction in cerebral blood flow.

## AIRWAY MANAGEMENT

Upper airway obstruction that cannot be relieved by other methods. Obstruction may be due to:
- laryngeal fracture
- edema of the glottis
- severe orofacial injuries
- severe oropharyngeal hemorrhage

## AIRWAY MANAGEMENT

Disadvantages of the nasopharyngeal airway (NPA) include:
- difficult to suction through
- does not isolate the trachea
- may be difficult to insert if nasal damage (new or old) is present.

## AIRWAY MANAGEMENT

- The narrowest part of the adult airway is at the vocal cords.
- The narrowest part of an infant's airway is at the cricoid ring.

## AIRWAY MANAGEMENT

Indications for use of the PtLA include:
- cardiac or respiratory arrest
- unconscious patient with suspected cervical spine injury
- unconscious patient in whom airway support or protection is needed
- unconscious patient in whom endotracheal intubation was unsuccessful

## AIRWAY MANAGEMENT

The EOA should not be used:
- in conscious patients
- for more than 2 hours
- in children under the age of 16
    - only available in one size
- in cases of known esophageal disease
- when caustic substances have been ingested

## AIRWAY MANAGEMENT

The proximal end of the endotracheal tube cuff should be advanced approximately 1-2.5 cm (1/2-1 inch) beyond the vocal cords.

## AIRWAY MANAGEMENT

When using a pocket mask, an oxygen flow rate of 10 liters/minute will provide an inspired oxygen concentration of approximately 50%.

## AIRWAY MANAGEMENT

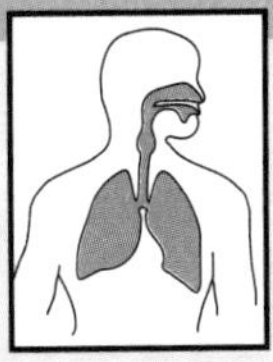

Name two advantages associated with the use of the oropharyngeal airway (OPA).

## AIRWAY MANAGEMENT

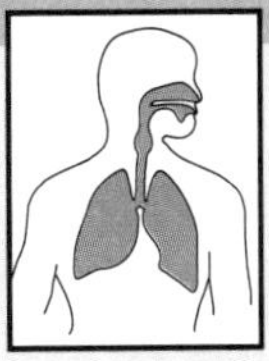

When is use of the pharyngotracheal lumen airway (PtLA) contraindicated?

## AIRWAY MANAGEMENT

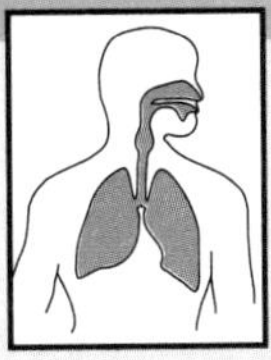

What is the purpose of the laryngoscope?

## AIRWAY MANAGEMENT

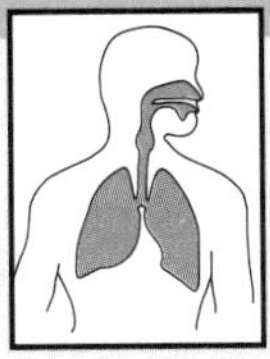

Name two indications for endotracheal intubation.

## AIRWAY MANAGEMENT

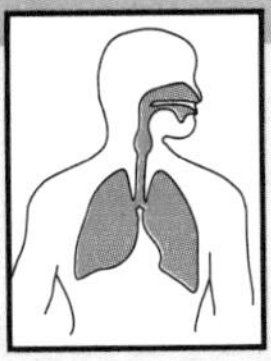

Describe an end-tidal CO2 detector.

## AIRWAY MANAGEMENT

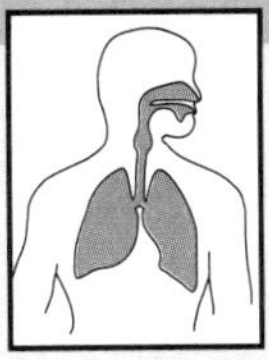

Name three patient conditions in which the value of pulse oximetry may be limited.

## AIRWAY MANAGEMENT

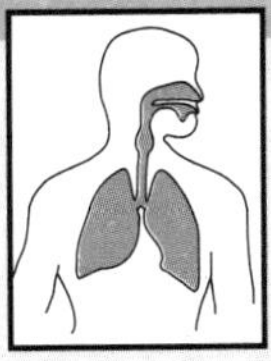

How is proper oropharyngeal airway (OPA) size determined?

## AIRWAY MANAGEMENT

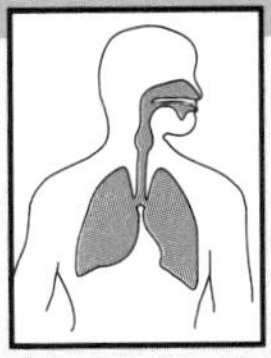

What is the most common problem associated with the use of the bag-valve-mask device?

## AIRWAY MANAGEMENT

The PtLA is contraindicated in:
- history of caustic ingestion
- patients less than 14 years of age
  - the PtLA is available in only one adult size
- known esophageal disease or injury
- conscious or semiconscious patients with an active gag reflex.

## AIRWAY MANAGEMENT

The oropharyngeal airway:
- permits suctioning on either side of the device
- holds the tongue away from the posterior wall of the pharynx
- may serve as an effective bite block in intubated patients, preventing biting of the endotracheal tube.

## AIRWAY MANAGEMENT

Indications for endotracheal intubation include:
- cardiac arrest with ongoing chest compressions
- inability of the conscious patient to ventilate adequately
- inability of the patient to protect his/her own airway (coma, areflexia, cardiac arrest)
- inability of the rescuer to ventilate the unconscious patient with conventional methods.

## AIRWAY MANAGEMENT

The laryngoscope:
- permits direct visualization of the vocal cords/glottis
- is used to align the structures of the upper airway to facilitate endotracheal intubation.

## AIRWAY MANAGEMENT

The value of pulse oximetry may be limited in:
- Anemia
- Hypothermia
- Cardiac arrest
- Peripheral edema
- Severe vascular disease
- Use of vasopressor therapy
- Carbon monoxide poisoning
- Hypotension (systolic BP < 50 mm Hg).

## AIRWAY MANAGEMENT

- The end-tidal CO2 detector is an instrument that attaches directly to an endotracheal tube between the ventilation device (bag-valve device or automatic transport ventilator) and the endotracheal tube.
- The end-tidal CO2 detector detects carbon dioxide in exhaled air..

## AIRWAY MANAGEMENT

The most common problem with the bag-valve-mask device is the inability to provide adequate ventilatory volume (in the non-intubated patient) due to the difficulty in providing a leakproof seal to the face while simultaneously maintaining an open airway.

## AIRWAY MANAGEMENT

- Place the oropharyngeal airway (OPA) against the patient's cheek with the flange of the OPA at the patient's lips.
- If the OPA is of proper size, the distal tip will reach the angle of the jaw.

## AIRWAY MANAGEMENT

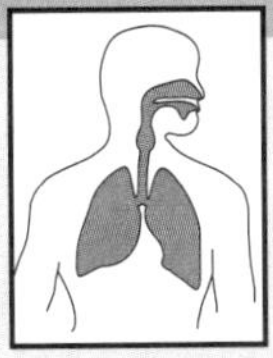

You have intubated a patient in cardiopulmonary arrest.

Name two possible consequences of unrecognized esophageal intubation.

## AIRWAY MANAGEMENT

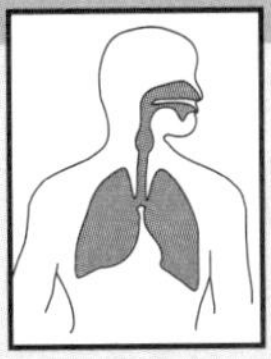

A 88 year old male is found unresponsive. Assessment reveals a carotid pulse is present but the victim is not breathing.

At what rate should rescue breathing be initiated?

## AIRWAY MANAGEMENT

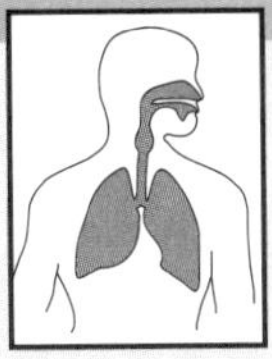

State the equipment needed for endotracheal intubation.

## AIRWAY MANAGEMENT

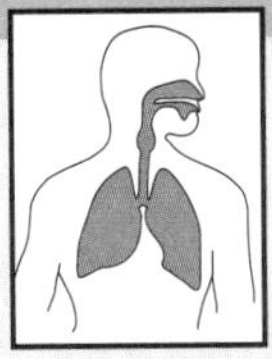

A 78 year old female has suffered a respiratory arrest. You have intubated the patient and note breath sounds are now present on the right but diminished on the left.

- What is the most likely cause of this situation?
- What corrective action will you initiate?

## AIRWAY MANAGEMENT

The American Heart Association recommends the delivery of one breath every 5-6 seconds (10-12 per minute).

## AIRWAY MANAGEMENT

- Cerebral hypoxia
- Brain damage
- Death

## AIRWAY MANAGEMENT

- The endotracheal tube is most likely in the right mainstem bronchus.
- Deflate the endotracheal tube cuff and pull back the tube slightly. Reinflate the endotracheal tube cuff and reassess breath sounds.

## AIRWAY MANAGEMENT

- Gloves, mask, protective eye wear
- Laryngoscope blade and handle
- Endotracheal tube (approximate size plus 1/2 size larger and 1/2 size smaller)
- Stylet
- 10 ml syringe
- Suction device
- Stethoscope
- Bag-valve device with reservoir and oxygen source
- Tape or other tube-securing device.

## DYSRHYTHMIA RECOGNITION

What is the normal duration of the PR interval?

## DYSRHYTHMIA RECOGNITION

What is the significance of the "absolute" refractory period?

## DYSRHYTHMIA RECOGNITION

What are the characteristics of first-degree AV block?

## DYSRHYTHMIA RECOGNITION

Identify the rhythm below.

Lead II

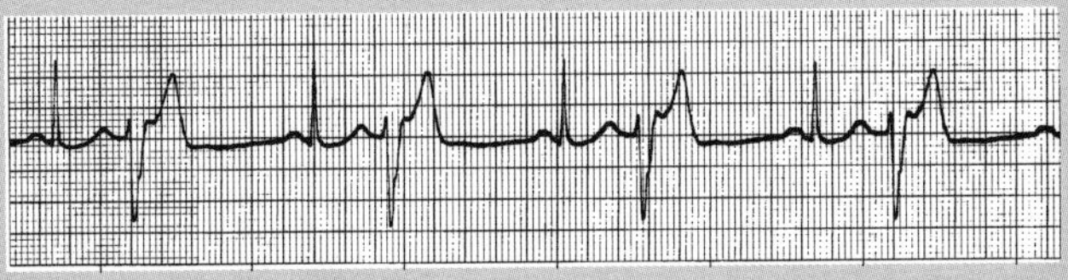

## DYSRHYTHMIA RECOGNITION

What are the characteristics of second-degree AV block, type I?

## DYSRHYTHMIA RECOGNITION

Name the two types of cardiac cells and describe their function.

## DYSRHYTHMIA RECOGNITION

Name the valve that separates the right ventricle from the right atrium.

## DYSRHYTHMIA RECOGNITION

Define "automaticity."

## DYSRHYTHMIA RECOGNITION

- The absolute refractory period (also known as the effective refractory period) extends from the onset of the QRS complex to approximately the peak of the T wave.
- During this period, cardiac cells have not yet repolarized and, no matter how strong a stimulus, cannot be stimulated to depolarize.

## DYSRHYTHMIA RECOGNITION

The PR interval normally measures 0.12 to 0.20 second.

## DYSRHYTHMIA RECOGNITION

The rhythm shown is a sinus bradycardia with ventricular bigeminy (every other beat is a premature ventricular complex).

## DYSRHYTHMIA RECOGNITION

Characteristics of first-degree AV block:

| | |
|---|---|
| Rate: | Atrial & ventricular within normal limits and the same |
| Rhythm: | Atrial & ventricular regular |
| P waves: | Normal in size and configuration; one P wave before each QRS |
| PR interval: | Prolonged (>.20 sec) but CONSTANT |
| QRS: | Usually 0.10 sec or less in duration |

## DYSRHYTHMIA RECOGNITION

- Myocardial (working) cells (also known as mechanical cells) are found in the myocardium. These cells contain contractile filaments that contract when the cells are electrically stimulated.
- Electrical (pacemaker) cells are found in the electrical conduction system. Their primary function is generation and conduction of electrical impulses.

## DYSRHYTHMIA RECOGNITION

Second-degree AV block, type I (Wenckebach, Mobitz I) is characterized by:

| | |
|---|---|
| Rate: | Atrial rate > ventricular rate; both are usually within normal limits |
| Rhythm: | Atrial regular (P's plot through); ventricular irregular |
| P waves: | Normal in size and configuration; some P waves are not followed by a QRS (more P's than QRS's) |
| PR interval: | Lengthens with each cycle (although lengthening may be slight) until a P wave appears without a QRS |
| QRS: | 0.10 sec or less in duration but is dropped periodically |

## DYSRHYTHMIA RECOGNITION

Automaticity refers to the ability of cardiac cells to spontaneously initiate an electrical impulse without being stimulated by an external source (such as a nerve).

## DYSRHYTHMIA RECOGNITION

The tricuspid valve separates the right atrium and right ventricle.

## DYSRHYTHMIA RECOGNITION

Identify the rhythm below.

Lead II

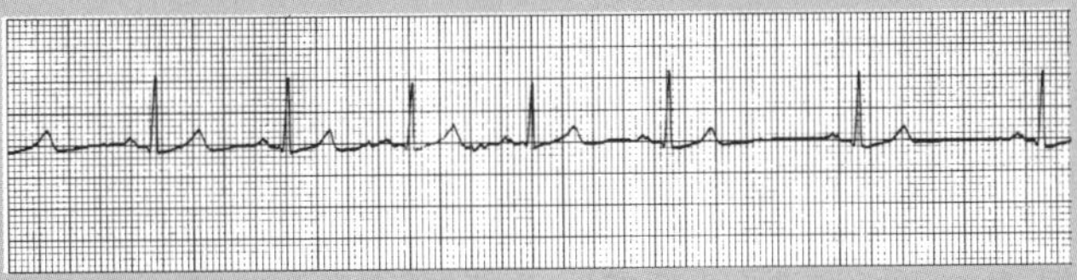

## DYSRHYTHMIA RECOGNITION

Identify the rhythm below.

Lead II

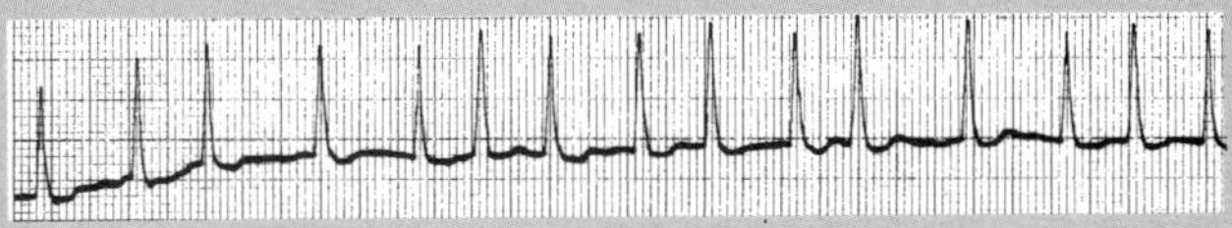

## DYSRHYTHMIA RECOGNITION

What is the normal pacemaker of the heart and where is it located?

## DYSRHYTHMIA RECOGNITION

Describe the primary function of the AV node.

## DYSRHYTHMIA RECOGNITION

State the inherent rate of the ventricles.

## DYSRHYTHMIA RECOGNITION

State the characteristics of atrial flutter.

## DYSRHYTHMIA RECOGNITION

Is depolarization the same as contraction?

## DYSRHYTHMIA RECOGNITION

Name the first positive deflection seen after the P wave on the ECG.

## DYSRHYTHMIA RECOGNITION

- The rhythm shown is atrial fibrillation with a rapid ventricular response.
- Characteristics of atrial fibrillation:

| | |
|---|---|
| Rate: | Atrial rate usually > 400, ventricular rate variable |
| Rhythm: | Atrial and ventricular very irregular |
| P waves: | No identifiable P waves; erratic, wavy baseline |
| PRI: | None |
| QRS: | Usually < 0.10 sec |

## DYSRHYTHMIA RECOGNITION

- The rhythm shown is a sinus arrhythmia.
- Characteristics of sinus arrhythmia:

| | |
|---|---|
| Rate: | Usually 60-100 beats/minute but may be faster or slower |
| Rhythm: | Irregular |
| P waves: | Uniform and upright in appearance; one preceding each QRS complex |
| PR interval: | 0.12-0.20 sec |
| QRS: | Usually 0.10 sec in duration or less |

## DYSRHYTHMIA RECOGNITION

- The main function of the atrio-ventricular (AV) node is to delay the electrical impulse.
- This allows the atria to contract and empty blood into the ventricles, promoting adequate ventricular filling before the next contraction of the ventricles.

## DYSRHYTHMIA RECOGNITION

- The normal pacemaker of the heart is the sino-atrial (SA) node because it depolarizes more rapidly than any other part of the cardiac conduction system.
- The SA node is located at the junction of the superior vena cava and the right atrium.

## DYSRHYTHMIA RECOGNITION

Characteristics of atrial flutter:

| | |
|---|---|
| Rate: | Atrial rate 250-350/minute; ventricular rate variable |
| Rhythm: | Atrial rhythm regular, ventricular rhythm usually regular but may be irregular |
| P waves: | Saw-toothed, "flutter waves" |
| PR interval: | Not measurable |
| QRS: | Usually 0.10 sec in duration or less but may be widened if flutter waves are buried in the QRS complex |

## DYSRHYTHMIA RECOGNITION

The inherent rate of the ventricles is 20 to 40 beats/minute.

## DYSRHYTHMIA RECOGNITION

The first positive deflection seen after the P wave on the ECG is the R wave.

## DYSRHYTHMIA RECOGNITION

- No. Depolarization is an electrical event, contraction is a mechanical event.
- We expect depolarization to result in stimulation of the myocardial working cells (mechanical cells) to contract, thus producing a pulse, however, it is possible for electrical activity to occur WITHOUT a mechanical response (pulse).
- When organized electrical activity with an adequate rate is viewed on the cardiac monitor and a pulse cannot be obtained, we term the clinical situation Pulseless Electrical Activity (PEA).

## DYSRHYTHMIA RECOGNITION

Identify the rhythm below.

Lead II

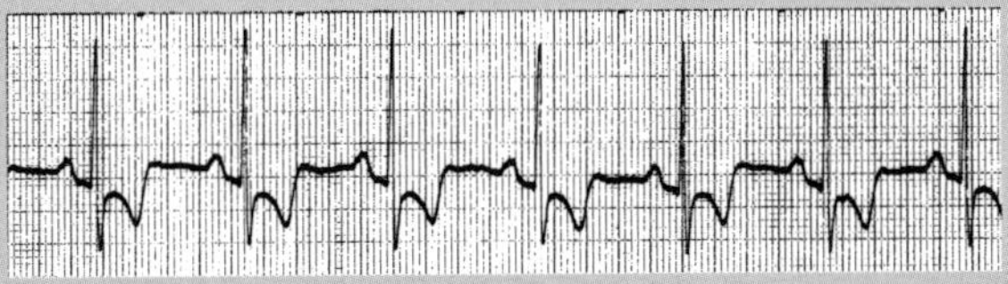

## DYSRHYTHMIA RECOGNITION

What is the significance of the relative refractory period?

## DYSRHYTHMIA RECOGNITION

Describe the PR interval in a junctional rhythm.

## DYSRHYTHMIA RECOGNITION

How would you determine if the ventricular rhythm on a rhythm strip was regular or irregular?

## DYSRHYTHMIA RECOGNITION

Identify the rhythm below.

Lead II

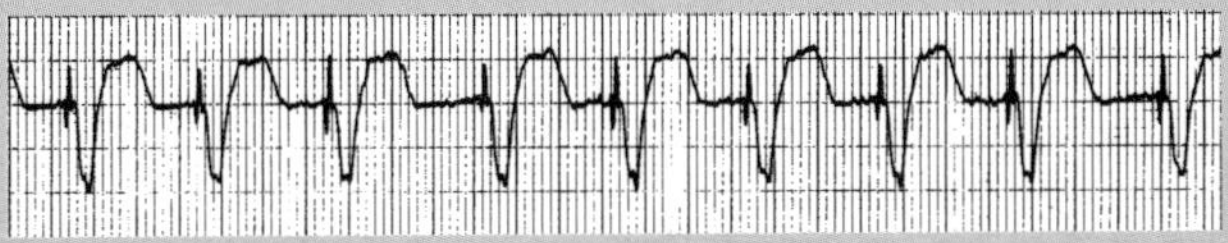

## DYSRHYTHMIA RECOGNITION

What is the AV junction?

## DYSRHYTHMIA RECOGNITION

What does the QRS complex represent?

## DYSRHYTHMIA RECOGNITION

Identify the rhythm below.

Lead II

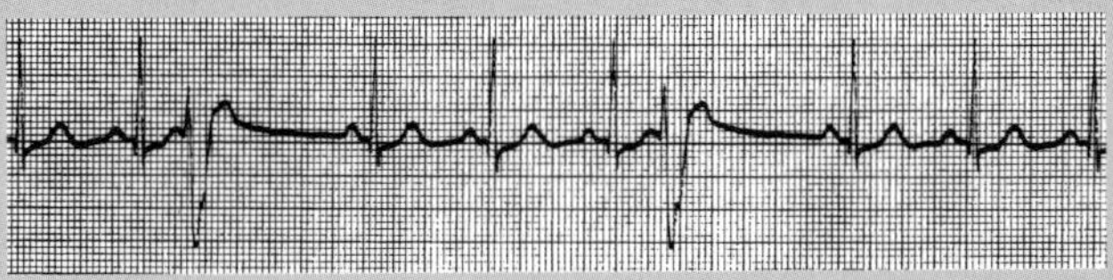

## DYSRHYTHMIA RECOGNITION

This is a 100% ventricular paced rhythm. Note the pacemaker spikes before each QRS complex.

## DYSRHYTHMIA RECOGNITION

The rhythm shown is a sinus rhythm with depressed ST segments and inverted T waves.

## DYSRHYTHMIA RECOGNITION

- The AV junction is the AV node and the non-branching portion of the bundle of His.
- The AV node does not contain pacemaker cells. The pacemaker cells in the AV junction are located near the nonbranching portion of the bundle of His.

## DYSRHYTHMIA RECOGNITION

- The relative refractory period (also known as the vulnerable period) corresponds with the downslope of the T wave.
- During this period most, but not all, cardiac cells have repolarized and can be stimulated to depolarize if a stimulus is strong enough.
- Should a stimulus precipitate depolarization during this period, chaos may result. For example, an R on T PVC may precipitate VT or VF.

## DYSRHYTHMIA RECOGNITION

The QRS complex represents ventricular depolarization.

## DYSRHYTHMIA RECOGNITION

- If the P wave precedes the QRS complex, the PR interval will be less than 0.12 second.
- If the P wave occurs during the QRS complex or after it, there will be no PR interval.

## DYSRHYTHMIA RECOGNITION

The rhythm shown is a sinus rhythm with two R on T premature ventricular complexes (PVCs).

## DYSRHYTHMIA RECOGNITION

- To determine if the ventricular rhythm is regular or irregular, measure the distance between two consecutive R-R intervals and compare that distance with another R-R interval.
- If the ventricular rhythm is regular, the R-R intervals will measure the same.

## DYSRHYTHMIA RECOGNITION

How is the PR interval measured?

## DYSRHYTHMIA RECOGNITION

Describe the location of the positive and negative electrodes in Lead I.

## DYSRHYTHMIA RECOGNITION

What does the QT interval represent and how is it measured?

## DYSRHYTHMIA RECOGNITION

How would you differentiate a junctional escape rhythm at 40 beats/minute from a ventricular escape rhythm at the same rate?

## DYSRHYTHMIA RECOGNITION

Identify the rhythm below.

Lead II

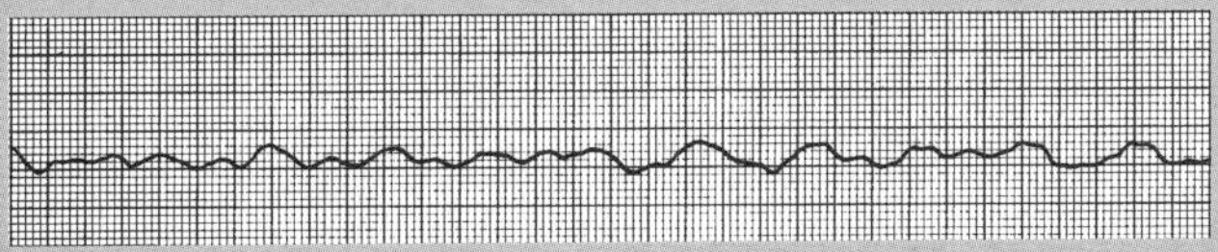

## DYSRHYTHMIA RECOGNITION

Describe an interpolated PVC.

## DYSRHYTHMIA RECOGNITION

Describe normal electrical flow through the heart.

## DYSRHYTHMIA RECOGNITION

State the inherent rate of the AV junction.

## DYSRHYTHMIA RECOGNITION

In Lead I:
- the positive electrode is placed just below the left clavicle
- the negative electrode is placed just below the right clavicle.

## DYSRHYTHMIA RECOGNITION

The PR interval is measured from the beginning of the P wave to the beginning of the QRS complex.

## DYSRHYTHMIA RECOGNITION

- A junctional escape rhythm is supraventricular in origin, thus it will have a narrow-QRS complex (.10 sec or less).
- A ventricular escape rhythm is ventricular in origin, thus it will have a wide-QRS complex (.12 second or greater).

## DYSRHYTHMIA RECOGNITION

- The QT interval represents total ventricular activity (the time required for ventricular depolarization and repolarization to take place).
- The QT interval is measured from the beginning of the QRS complex to the end of the T wave.

## DYSRHYTHMIA RECOGNITION

An interpolated PVC occurs between two normal beats and does not interrupt the underlying rhythm.

## DYSRHYTHMIA RECOGNITION

The rhythm shown is ventricular fibrillation.

## DYSRHYTHMIA RECOGNITION

The inherent rate of the AV junction is 40-60 beats/minute.

## DYSRHYTHMIA RECOGNITION

The impulse originates in the SA node and travels to the AV node, to the bundle of His, to the left and right bundle branches, to the Purkinje fibers where the mechanical cells are stimulated.

## DYSRHYTHMIA RECOGNITION

State the characteristics of third-degree (complete) AV block.

## DYSRHYTHMIA RECOGNITION

Describe the appearance of Torsades de Pointes.

## DYSRHYTHMIA RECOGNITION

What is the normal rate range of a sinus tachycardia?

## DYSRHYTHMIA RECOGNITION

What is the normal duration of the QRS complex in the adult?

## DYSRHYTHMIA RECOGNITION

Describe the PR intervals in the patient with a second-degree AV block, type I and the patient with a second-degree AV block, type II.

## DYSRHYTHMIA RECOGNITION

Where is the level of AV block in:

- Second-degree AV block, Type I?
- Second-degree AV block, Type II?

## DYSRHYTHMIA RECOGNITION

Indicate the correct position for the positive and negative electrodes in Lead $MCL_1$.

## DYSRHYTHMIA RECOGNITION

How would you determine if the atrial rhythm on a rhythm strip was regular or irregular?

## DYSRHYTHMIA RECOGNITION

- Torsades de Pointes is a type of polymorphic ventricular tachycardia characterized by a ventricular rate between 150 and 250 beats/minute and a gradual alteration in the amplitude and direction of the QRS ("twisting of the points").
- The QRS measures > .12 second.

## DYSRHYTHMIA RECOGNITION

Third-degree (complete) AV block:

- More P waves than QRS complexes
- P waves occur regularly
- Regular ventricular rhythm
- No PR interval because the atria and ventricles beat independently of each other
- QRS may be wide or narrow depending on the location of the escape pacemaker and the condition of the interventricular conduction system.

## DYSRHYTHMIA RECOGNITION

The normal duration of the QRS complex in the adult is 0.04 to 0.10 second.

## DYSRHYTHMIA RECOGNITION

The rate of a sinus tachycardia is normally 100-160 beats/minute.

## DYSRHYTHMIA RECOGNITION

- Second-degree AV block, Type I (Wenckebach, Mobitz I) almost always occurs at the level of the AV node.
  - narrow-QRS
- Second-degree AV block, Type II (Mobitz II) usually occurs at or below the bundle of His.
  - wide-QRS

## DYSRHYTHMIA RECOGNITION

- In second-degree AV block, type I (Wenckebach, Mobitz I), the PR intervals lengthen until a P wave appears without a QRS.
- In second-degree AV block, type II (Mobitz II), the PR interval may be normal or prolonged, but will measure the same for each conducted QRS.

## DYSRHYTHMIA RECOGNITION

- To determine if the atrial rhythm is regular or irregular, measure the distance between two consecutive P-P intervals and compare that distance with another P-P interval.
- If the atrial rhythm is regular, the P-P intervals will measure the same.

## DYSRHYTHMIA RECOGNITION

In Lead $MCL_1$:

- the negative electrode is placed just below the left clavicle
- the positive electrode is placed to the right of the sternum at the fourth intercostal space.

## DYSRHYTHMIA RECOGNITION

Name three possible causes of sinus tachycardia.

## DYSRHYTHMIA RECOGNITION

State the inherent rate of the SA node.

## DYSRHYTHMIA RECOGNITION

Describe correct placement of the positive and negative electrodes in Lead III.

## DYSRHYTHMIA RECOGNITION

Define the terms "dysrhythmia" and "arrhythmia."

## DYSRHYTHMIA RECOGNITION

Describe the appearance of second-degree AV block, 2:1 conduction on the cardiac monitor.

## DYSRHYTHMIA RECOGNITION

What is the action potential?

## DYSRHYTHMIA RECOGNITION

What is meant by the term "agonal rhythm"?

## DYSRHYTHMIA RECOGNITION

Name five basic steps used in analyzing a rhythm strip.

## DYSRHYTHMIA RECOGNITION

The inherent rate of the SA node is 60 to 100 beats/minute.

## DYSRHYTHMIA RECOGNITION

Possible causes of sinus tachycardia include (among many others):

- fever
- pain
- stress
- anxiety
- hypoxia
- pump failure
- compensatory response in shock

## DYSRHYTHMIA RECOGNITION

- The term "dysrhythmia" means abnormal rhythm.
- The term "arrhythmia" means absence of rhythm.
- Although there is a technical difference in the meaning of these terms, they are used interchangeably.

## DYSRHYTHMIA RECOGNITION

In Lead III:

- The positive electrode is placed just below the left pectoral muscle
- The negative electrode is placed just below the left clavicle.

## DYSRHYTHMIA RECOGNITION

- Electrical impulses occur as the result of brief but rapid flow of positively charged ions back and forth across the cell membrane.
- The cardiac action potential is an illustration of the changes in the membrane potential of a cardiac cell during depolarization and repolarization.

## DYSRHYTHMIA RECOGNITION

Second-degree AV block, 2:1 conduction:

- More P waves than QRS complexes
- P waves occur regularly
- Every other P wave is followed by a QRS
- The PR interval is CONSTANT
- The QRS may be WIDE or NARROW
    - Narrow if the block occurs above the bundle of His (probably second-degree AV block, type I)
    - Wide if the block occurs at or below the bundle of His (probably second-degree AV block, type II)

## DYSRHYTHMIA RECOGNITION

1. Rate
2. Rhythm
3. P waves
    - upright or inverted?
    - uniform in appearance?
    - one P wave before each QRS?
    - do the P waves occur regularly?
4. PR interval
    - duration?
5. QRS complexes
    - wide or narrow?

## DYSRHYTHMIA RECOGNITION

An agonal rhythm is also known as "dying heart" and is used to describe a rhythm similar in appearance to a ventricular escape rhythm except the rate is less than 20 beats per minute.

## DYSRHYTHMIA RECOGNITION

Describe the appearance of atrial activity in atrial fibrillation on the ECG.

## DYSRHYTHMIA RECOGNITION

Identify the rhythm below.

Lead II

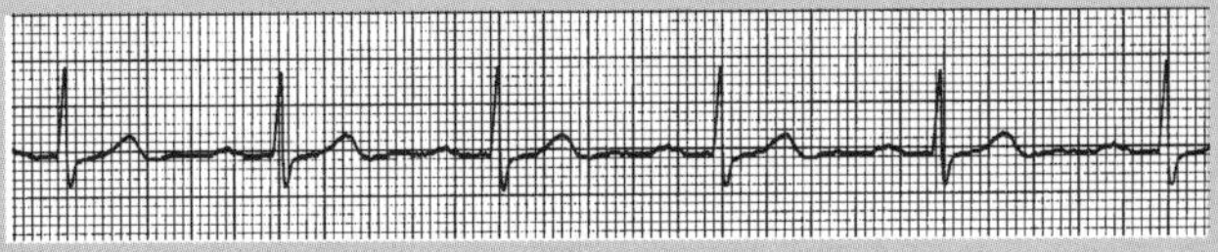

## DYSRHYTHMIA RECOGNITION

Describe the rhythm of a sinus arrhythmia.

## DYSRHYTHMIA RECOGNITION

Identify the rhythm below.

Lead II

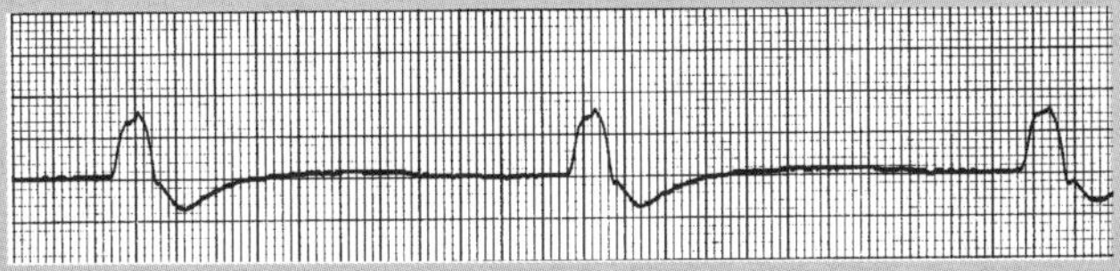

## DYSRHYTHMIA RECOGNITION

What portion of the ECG represents ventricular repolarization?

## DYSRHYTHMIA RECOGNITION

What is meant by the terms "controlled" and "uncontrolled" atrial fibrillation?

## DYSRHYTHMIA RECOGNITION

How does complete (third-degree) AV block differ from second-degree AV block, type I?

## DYSRHYTHMIA RECOGNITION

Second-degree AV block, type I is also known by two other names. What are they?

## DYSRHYTHMIA RECOGNITION

- The rhythm shown is a sinus rhythm with a first degree AV block.
- Characteristics of first-degree AV block:

| | |
|---|---|
| Rate: | Atrial and ventricular rates with normal limits |
| Rhythm: | Atrial and ventricular regular |
| P waves: | Normal in size and configuration; one P wave for each QRS |
| PR interval: | Prolonged (> 0.20 sec) but constant |
| QRS: | < 0.10 sec |

## DYSRHYTHMIA RECOGNITION

In atrial fibrillation, the atria are not contracting, they are quivering. This produces an erratic, wavy baseline (fibrillatory waves, f waves) on the ECG. P waves are not visible.

## DYSRHYTHMIA RECOGNITION

- The rhythm shown is an idioventricular (ventricular escape) rhythm.
- Characteristics of an idioventricular rhythm:

| | |
|---|---|
| Rate: | Atrial not discernible; ventricular 20-40 beats/minute |
| Rhythm: | Atrial not discernible; ventricular essentially regular |
| P waves: | Absent |
| PRI: | None |
| QRS: | > 0.12 sec |

## DYSRHYTHMIA RECOGNITION

The rhythm increases with inspiration and decreases with expiration.

## DYSRHYTHMIA RECOGNITION

- Atrial fibrillation with a ventricular response of less than 100 beats/minute is termed "controlled" atrial fibrillation.
- Atrial fibrillation with a ventricular response greater than 100 beats/minute is termed "uncontrolled" atrial fibrillation.

## DYSRHYTHMIA RECOGNITION

The T wave represents ventricular repolarization.

## DYSRHYTHMIA RECOGNITION

Second-degree AV block, type I is also known as:

- Wenckebach
- Mobitz I

## DYSRHYTHMIA RECOGNITION

- In complete (third-degree) AV block:
  - there is a regular atrial and ventricular rhythm
  - there is no PR interval since the atria and ventricles beat independently of each other.
- In second-degree AV block, type I (Wenckebach):
  - the atrial rhythm is regular
  - the ventricular rhythm is irregular
  - the PR interval lengthens until a P wave appears with no QRS.

## DYSRHYTHMIA RECOGNITION

Describe two methods for calculation of heart rate.

## DYSRHYTHMIA RECOGNITION

Name three possible causes of premature atrial complexes (PACs).

## DYSRHYTHMIA RECOGNITION

If the QRS measures 0.10 second or less, it is presumed to be ____ in origin.

## DYSRHYTHMIA RECOGNITION

What is the significance of a PR interval measuring less than 0.12 or more than 0.20 second?

## DYSRHYTHMIA RECOGNITION

Identify the rhythm below.

Lead II

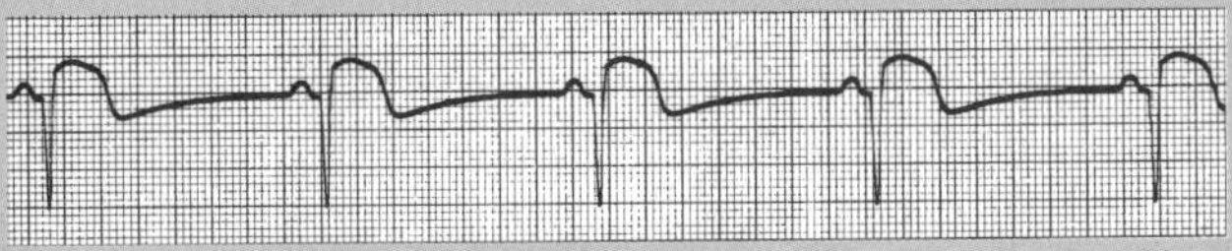

## DYSRHYTHMIA RECOGNITION

Identify the rhythm below.

Lead II

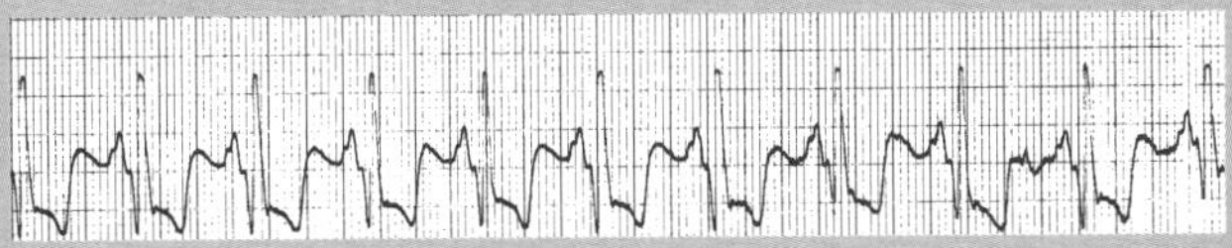

## DYSRHYTHMIA RECOGNITION

Identify the rhythm below.

Lead II

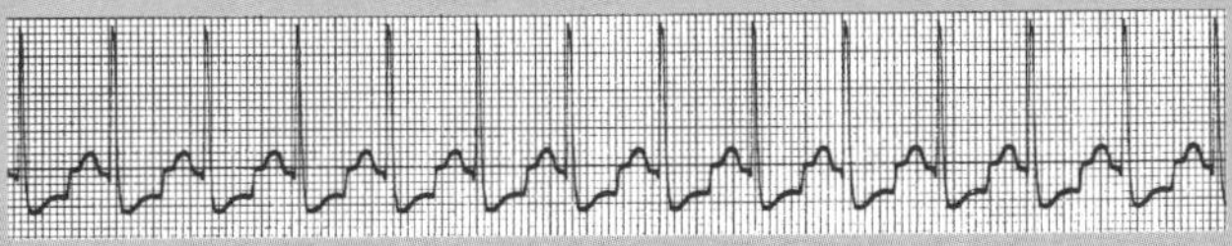

## DYSRHYTHMIA RECOGNITION

Identify the rhythm below.

Lead II

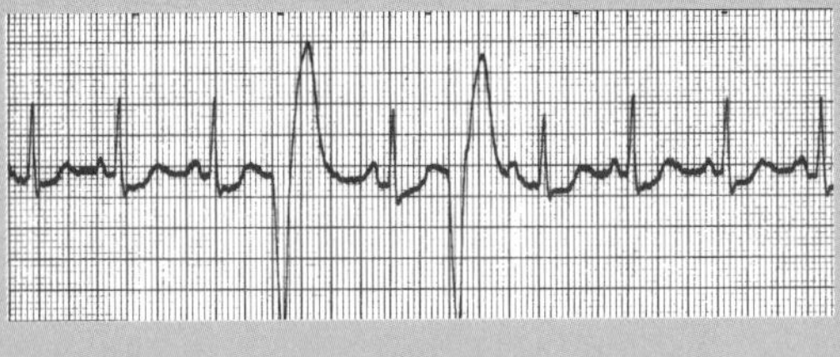

## DYSRHYTHMIA RECOGNITION

- The rhythm is a sinus bradycardia with elevated ST segments.
- Characteristics of this dysrhythmia:

| | |
|---|---|
| Rate: | <60 beats/minute |
| Rhythm: | Atrial and ventricular rhythm regular |
| P waves: | Uniform and upright; one P wave before each QRS |
| PR interval: | 0.12-0.20 sec |
| QRS: | Usually 0.10 second or less in duration. |

## DYSRHYTHMIA RECOGNITION

- Each small square represents 0.04 sec on ECG paper. There are 1500 boxes in one minute. To determine ventricular rate, count the number of small squares between two consecutive R waves and divide into 1500.
- Count the number of large squares (5 small boxes) between two R waves and divide into 300.
- Count the number of complete R waves with a period of 6 seconds and multiply that number by 10 to determine the rate for one minute.

## DYSRHYTHMIA RECOGNITION

The rhythm shown is a sinus rhythm (borderline sinus tachycardia).

- Note the significant Q waves, depressed ST segments and inverted T waves.

## DYSRHYTHMIA RECOGNITION

- Often unknown
- Hypoxia
- Digitalis toxicity
- Sympathomimetic drugs
- Congestive heart failure
- Myocardial ischemia or injury
- Use of stimulants (excess coffee, tobacco, alcohol)

## DYSRHYTHMIA RECOGNITION

- The rhythm shown is a sinus tachycardia with depressed ST segments and inverted T waves.
- Characteristics of a sinus tachycardia:

| | |
|---|---|
| Rate: | 100-160 beats/minute |
| Rhythm: | Regular |
| P waves: | Uniform and upright in appearance<br>One preceding each QRS complex |
| PR interval: | 0.12-0.20 sec |
| QRS: | 0.10 sec in duration or less |

## DYSRHYTHMIA RECOGNITION

If the QRS measures 0.10 second or less (narrow), it is presumed to be SUPRAventricular in origin.

## DYSRHYTHMIA RECOGNITION

The rhythm shown is a sinus rhythm with frequent, uniform premature ventricular complexes (PVCs).

## DYSRHYTHMIA RECOGNITION

If the PR interval measures less than 0.12 or more than 0.20 second, conduction followed an abnormal pathway or the impulse was delayed in the area of the AV node.

## DYSRHYTHMIA RECOGNITION

Identify the rhythm below.

Lead II

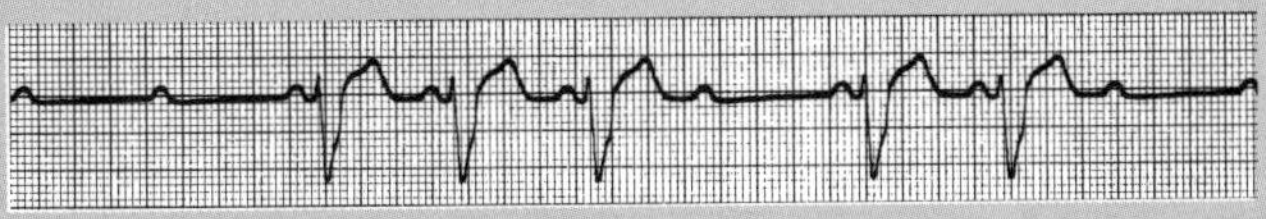

## DYSRHYTHMIA RECOGNITION

Identify the rhythm below.

Lead II

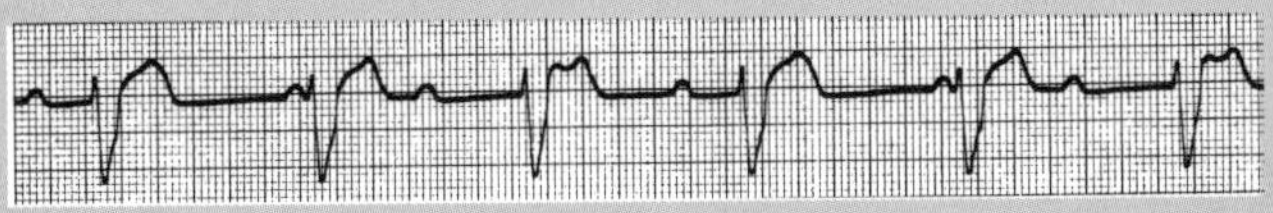

## DYSRHYTHMIA RECOGNITION

Identify the rhythm below.

Lead II

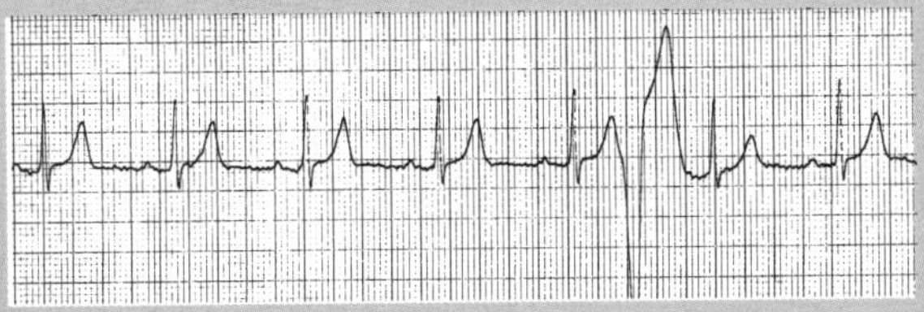

## DYSRHYTHMIA RECOGNITION

Identify the rhythm below.

Lead II

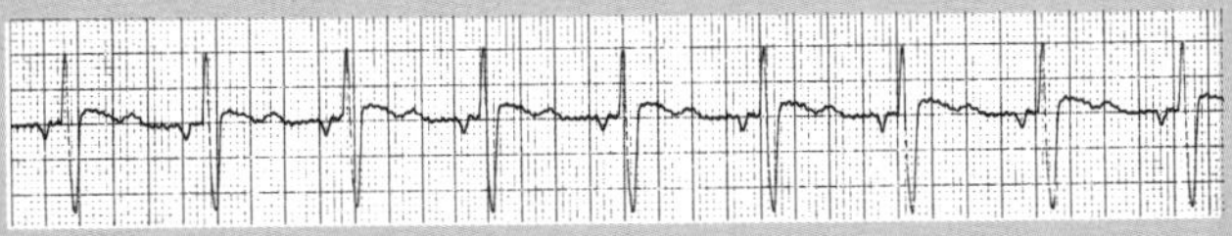

## DYSRHYTHMIA RECOGNITION

Name two possible causes of an accelerated junctional rhythm.

## DYSRHYTHMIA RECOGNITION

Identify the rhythm below.

Lead II

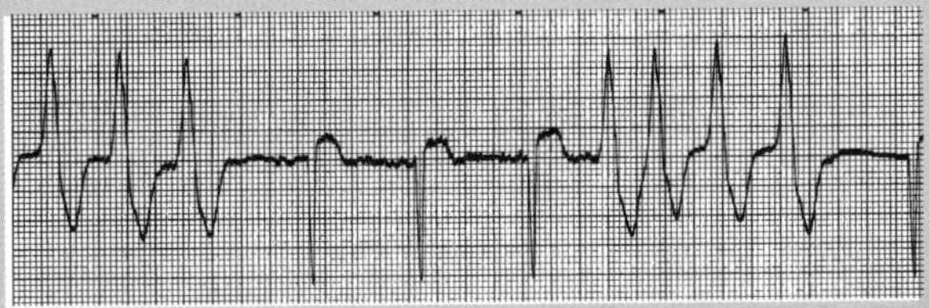

## DYSRHYTHMIA RECOGNITION

Name the ECG changes commonly seen in cases of hyperkalemia.

## DYSRHYTHMIA RECOGNITION

Name two possible mechanisms of cardiac dysrhythmias.

## DYSRHYTHMIA RECOGNITION

- The rhythm is a complete (third-degree) AV block.
- Characteristics of complete AV block:

Rate: Atrial rate > ventricular rate; ventricular rate determined by the origin of the escape rhythm
Rhythm: Atrial regular (P's plot through); ventricular regular
P waves: More P's than QRS's
PR interval: None - the atria and ventricles beat independently of each other; no relationship between the P's and QRS's
QRS: May be wide or narrow depending on the location of the escape pacemaker and the condition of the interventricular conduction system. Narrow = junctional pacemaker; wide = ventricular pacemaker.

## DYSRHYTHMIA RECOGNITION

- The rhythm shown is second-degree AV block type II.
- Second-degree AV block, type II is characterized by:

Rate: Atrial rate > ventricular rate
Rhythm: Atrial regular (P's plot through); ventricular irregular
P waves: Normal in size and configuration; some P waves are not followed by a QRS (more P's than QRS's)
PR interval: May be within normal limits or prolonged but is CONSTANT FOR EACH CONDUCTED QRS
QRS: >0.10 sec but is dropped periodically.

## DYSRHYTHMIA RECOGNITION

- The rhythm shown is an accelerated junctional rhythm.
- An accelerated junctional rhythm is characterized by:

Rate: 60-100 beats/minute
Rhythm: Atrial and ventricular very regular
P waves: May occur before, during or after the QRS; if seen (as shown in this example), will be inverted (retrograde)
PR interval: Not measurable unless the P wave precedes the QRS; when present, will usually be less than or equal to 0.12 sec
QRS: 0.10 sec or less

## DYSRHYTHMIA RECOGNITION

The rhythm shown is a sinus rhythm with an R on T interpolated premature ventricular complex.

- The premature ventricular complex is termed R on T because the premature beat occurs before the T wave of the sinus beat returns to the baseline.
- The premature complex is also termed an interpolated PVC because the beat occurs between to normal beats and does not interrupt the underlying sinus rhythm.

## DYSRHYTHMIA RECOGNITION

The rhythm displayed is atrial fibrillation with two runs of ventricular tachycardia.

- Three or more sequential premature ventricular complexes (PVCs) are referred to as a run, burst or salvo of ventricular tachycardia.

## DYSRHYTHMIA RECOGNITION

An accelerated junctional rhythm is commonly seen in patients with digitalis toxicity. This rhythm may also occur as a result of inferior wall MI or post open heart surgery.

## DYSRHYTHMIA RECOGNITION

Cardiac dysrhythmias may result from:

1. Disturbances in automaticity
   - Sinus bradycardia or sinus tachycardia
   - Premature atrial, junctional or ventricular complexes
   - Atrial or ventricular tachycardia
2. Disturbances in conductivity
   - Wolff-Parkinson-White syndrome
   - AV block
3. Combinations of altered automaticity or conductivity
   - First degree AV block with premature atrial complexes

## DYSRHYTHMIA RECOGNITION

ECG changes progress as the potassium level rises:

- Potassium level between 6.5 and 7.5 mEq/L
  - Prolonging PR interval, widening of the QRS complex, decrease in P wave amplitude, ST segment elevation or depression, tall peaked T waves
- Potassium level between 7.5 and 8.5 mEq/L
  - Further widening of the QRS, flattening and widening of the P wave, AV block and bundle branch blocks may occur
- Potassium level greater than 8.5 mEq/L
  - Absent P wave, further widening of the QRS, ventricular dysrhythmias (including VT, VF, asystole).

## DYSRHYTHMIA RECOGNITION

A conduction problem above the level of the bundle branches will largely affect which portions of the cardiac cycle?

## DYSRHYTHMIA RECOGNITION

What is meant by the term "blocked" or "nonconducted" premature atrial complex?

## DYSRHYTHMIA RECOGNITION

Describe the significance of a negative P wave in Lead II.

## DYSRHYTHMIA RECOGNITION

When is the term "supraventricular tachycardia" used?

## DYSRHYTHMIA RECOGNITION

Why is the term premature ventricular complex more correct than premature ventricular contraction?

## DYSRHYTHMIA RECOGNITION

Name two possible causes of Torsades de Pointes.

## DYSRHYTHMIA RECOGNITION

Is the QRS complex wide or narrow in third-degree (complete) AV block?

## DYSRHYTHMIA RECOGNITION

Name two possible causes of complete (third-degree) AV block.

## DYSRHYTHMIA RECOGNITION

- When a premature atrial complex (PAC) occurs very early and close to the preceding beat, a P wave may be seen with no QRS complex after it ("blocked" or "nonconducted" PAC).
- This occurs because the premature P wave occurred so early the ventricles were still refractory and unable to conduct the impulse (thus, no QRS complex).

## DYSRHYTHMIA RECOGNITION

- A conduction problem above the level of the bundle branches will largely affect the P wave and the PR interval.
- A conduction problem below this point will largely affect the QRS complex.

## DYSRHYTHMIA RECOGNITION

- Supraventricular tachycardia (SVT) is not a specific dysrhythmia but is a term used to describe a rhythm that cannot be distinguished from another with similar characteristics at the same rate. For example, the following dysrhythmias possess overlapping rate ranges:

| | |
|---|---|
| Atrial flutter | 150-250 beats/minute |
| Atrial tachycardia | 150-250 beats/minute |
| Junctional tach | 100-180 beats/minute |

- SVT is characterized by a regular ventricular rhythm with a narrow-QRS complex in which P waves cannot be distinguished from the preceding T wave.

## DYSRHYTHMIA RECOGNITION

If the P wave is negative in Lead II, the impulse most likely began in or near the AV junction and was conducted away from the area of the AV junction backward toward the SA node (retrograde conduction).

## DYSRHYTHMIA RECOGNITION

1. Drug induced
    - Cyclic antidepressants (doxepin, imipramine, amitriptyline)
    - Phenothiazines (Haloperidol, Chlorpromazine, Thioridazine)
    - Type I antidysrhythmics (quinidine, procainamide, disopyramide, tocainaide, mexiletine)
2. Eating disorders (bulimia, anorexia)
3. Electrolyte abnormalities
    - Hypomagnesemia
    - Hypokalemia
    - Hypocalcemia

## DYSRHYTHMIA RECOGNITION

- The ECG is a representation of electrical activity.
- The term premature ventricular contraction implies mechanical activity occurred which cannot be determined unless the patient's pulse is assessed.
- Premature ventricular complex is the more correct term.

## DYSRHYTHMIA RECOGNITION

Possible causes of complete (third-degree) AV block include:

- ischemia
- rheumatic fever
- digitalis toxicity
- congenital abnormalities
- acute anterior MI (usually wide QRS)
- acute inferior MI (usually narrow QRS)
- extensive conduction system disease

## DYSRHYTHMIA RECOGNITION

The QRS complex may be either wide or narrow in a third-degree (complete) AV block.

- The QRS will be narrow if a junctional escape rhythm is present.
- The QRS will be wide if a ventricular escape rhythm is present.

## DYSRHYTHMIA RECOGNITION

Name two ECG changes that may be seen with hypomagnesemia.

## DYSRHYTHMIA RECOGNITION

Identify the rhythm below.

Lead II

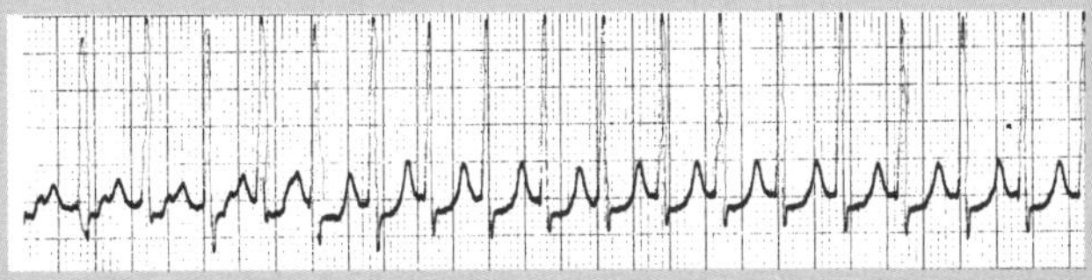

## DYSRHYTHMIA RECOGNITION

What is multifocal atrial tachycardia?

## DYSRHYTHMIA RECOGNITION

Identify the rhythm below.

Lead II

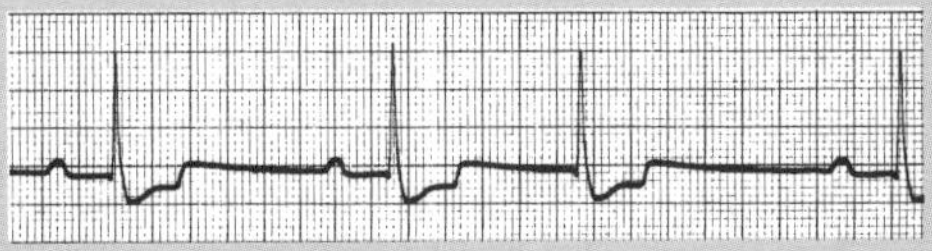

## DYSRHYTHMIA RECOGNITION

What is Wolff-Parkinson-White Syndrome?

## DYSRHYTHMIA RECOGNITION

Name two possible causes of second-degree AV block, type I.

## DYSRHYTHMIA RECOGNITION

Explain the difference between a premature ventricular complex and a ventricular escape beat.

## DYSRHYTHMIA RECOGNITION

State the characteristics of a supraventricular tachycardia.

## DYSRHYTHMIA RECOGNITION

The rhythm displayed is a sinus tachycardia with a premature atrial complex which precipitates paroxysmal (sudden onset) supraventricular tachycardia (PSVT).

## DYSRHYTHMIA RECOGNITION

ECG changes seen with hypomagnesemia are similar to those seen with hypokalemia.

- Prolonged PR intervals
- ST segment depression
- Flattened T waves

## DYSRHYTHMIA RECOGNITION

The rhythm shown is sinus bradycardia with a first degree AV block and a premature junctional complex (PJC). Note the presence of ST segment depression and inverted T waves.

- The first degree AV block is identified by the prolonged PR interval (> 0.20 sec).
- The premature junction complex is the third complex from the left identified by its narrow QRS and absent P wave.

## DYSRHYTHMIA RECOGNITION

- Multifocal atrial tachycardia is also known as chaotic atrial tachycardia. This rhythm frequently precedes the onset of atrial fibrillation and may be due to hypoxia, electrolyte imbalance or chronic pulmonary disease.
- Multifocal atrial tachycardia is characterized by:

| | |
|---|---|
| Rate: | Greater than 100 beats/minute |
| Rhythm: | Atrial and ventricular rhythms are irregular |
| PR interval: | May be normal or vary |
| P waves: | Three or more differently shaped P waves |
| QRS: | Within normal limits |

## DYSRHYTHMIA RECOGNITION

Possible causes of second-degree AV block, type I include:

- rheumatic fever
- digitalis toxicity
- inferior wall MI or ischemia
- increased parasympathetic tone
- drug therapy (propranolol, verapamil, digitalis)

## DYSRHYTHMIA RECOGNITION

- WPW is the most common type of pre-excitation syndrome. In patients with WPW, a bundle of working myocardial tissue forms a connection between the atria and ventricles outside the normal conduction system (referred to as an accessory pathway). This pathway may connect the right atrial and ventricular walls, the left atrial and ventricular walls or connect the atrial and ventricular septa on either the right or left side.
- The accessory pathway conducts faster than the AV node (where impulses are normally delayed). The PR interval in WPW is short since there is no delay in the accessory pathway. The QRS is often > 0.10 sec and recognized by a slurring of the beginning of the QRS complex (the delta wave) because the ventricles are pre-excited by the impulse which originated outside of the normal conduction system.

## DYSRHYTHMIA RECOGNITION

Supraventricular tachycardia is characterized by:

| | |
|---|---|
| Rate: | Ventricular 150-250 beats/minute |
| Rhythm: | Regular ventricular rhythm |
| P waves: | Usually identifiable at the lower end of this rate range but are seldom identifiable at rates greater than 200 beats/minute |
| PR interval: | Often not measurable because the P wave is difficult to distinguish from the preceding T wave; if measurable, is 0.12-0.20 sec |
| QRS: | 0.10 sec or less in duration |

## DYSRHYTHMIA RECOGNITION

- A premature ventricular complex is, by definition, premature, occurring earlier than the next expected beat.
- Ventricular escape beats occur late in the cardiac cycle, occurring after the next expected beat.
    - Ventricular escape beats are protective.
- Although lidocaine may be indicated for significant PVCs in the setting of acute MI, lidocaine should NOT be administered for escape beats.

## DYSRHYTHMIA RECOGNITION

Identify the rhythm below.

Lead II

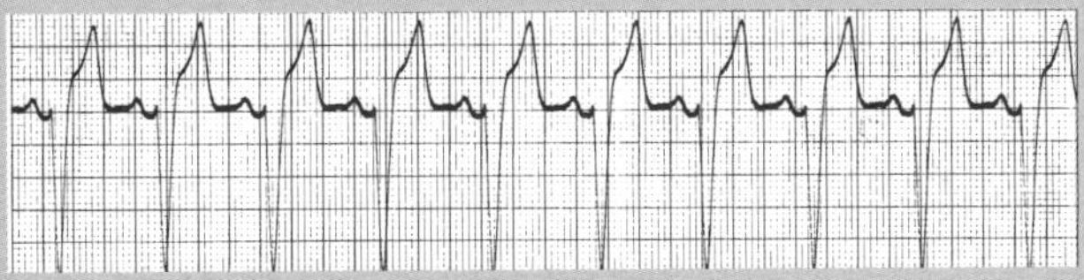

## DYSRHYTHMIA RECOGNITION

Identify the rhythm below.

Lead II

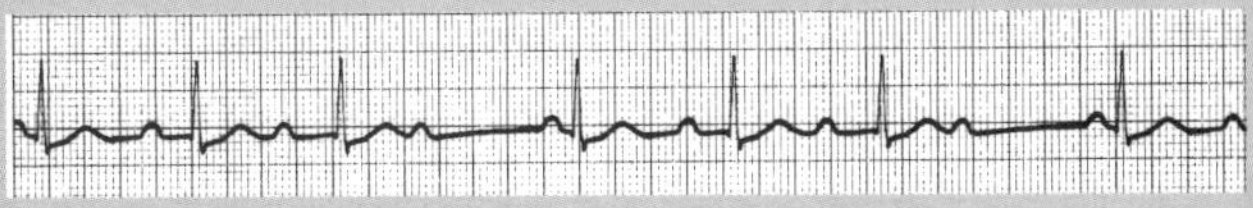

## DYSRHYTHMIA RECOGNITION

- The rhythm is second-degree AV block type I.
- Characteristics of this dysrhythmia:

| | |
|---|---|
| Rate: | Atrial rate > ventricular rate, both are usually within normal limits |
| Rhythm: | Atrial rhythm regular (P waves plot through); ventricular rhythm irregular |
| P waves: | Normal in size and configuration; some P waves are not followed by a QRS (more Pís than QRSís) |
| PR interval: | Lengthens with each cycle until a P wave appears without a QRS |
| QRS: | 0.10 sec or less but is dropped periodically |

## DYSRHYTHMIA RECOGNITION

The rhythm shown is a sinus rhythm with elevated ST segments.

## ELECTRICAL THERAPY

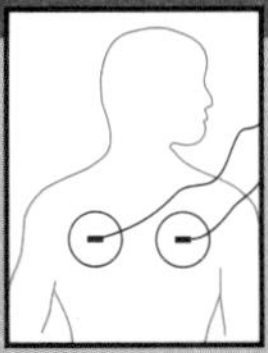

Name four possibilities to consider if the cardiac monitor displays a flat line.

## ELECTRICAL THERAPY

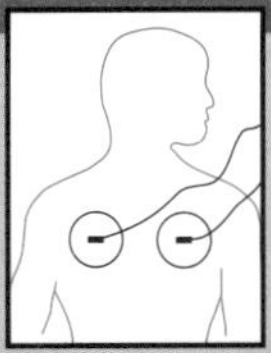

Name two indications for the delivery of unsynchronized countershock.

## ELECTRICAL THERAPY

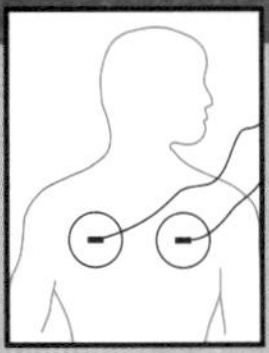

Management of unstable patients may necessitate the use of electrical therapy.

Identify the correct energy settings for management of an unstable patient with atrial flutter.

## ELECTRICAL THERAPY

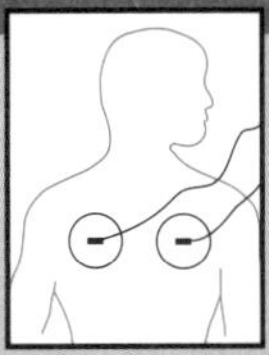

Identify the correct energy settings for management of the unstable patient in monomorphic ventricular tachycardia (VT).

## ELECTRICAL THERAPY

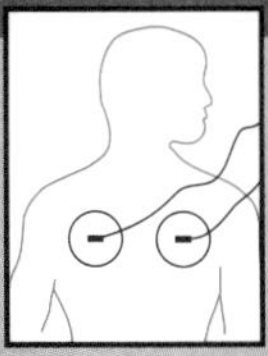

Name two possible complications of transcutaneous pacing.

## ELECTRICAL THERAPY

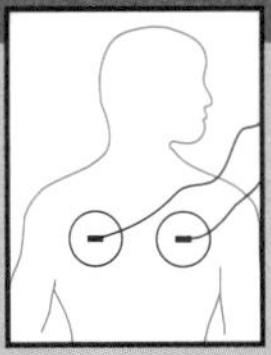

A 75 year old female has suffered a cardiac arrest. You have applied conventional defibrillator paddles to the chest for a "quick-look." The cardiac monitor displays asystole. You recall that you should confirm this rhythm in another lead.

Using the quick-look paddles, how will you do this?

## ELECTRICAL THERAPY

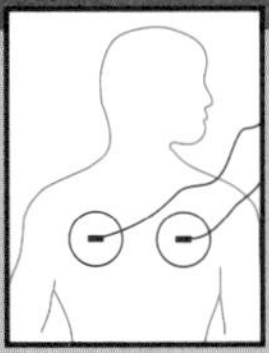

Name four factors that affect transthoracic resistance.

## ELECTRICAL THERAPY

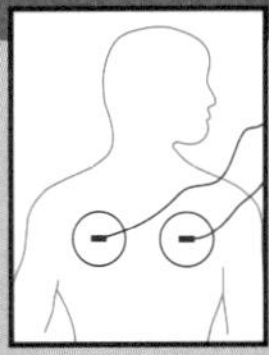

Management of unstable patients may necessitate the use of electrical therapy.

Identify the correct energy settings for management of an unstable patient with atrial fibrillation.

## ELECTRICAL THERAPY

Unsynchronized countershock is indicated:
- in ventricular fibrillation (VF)
- in sustained Torsades de Pointes
- in pulseless ventricular tachycardia (VT)
- in ventricular tachycardia with a pulse if there is an undue delay in synchronization or if the patient's clinical condition is critical.

## ELECTRICAL THERAPY

Possibilities include:
- no power
- loose leads
- true asystole
- isoelectric VF/VT
- no connection to the patient
- no connection to the defibrillator/monitor

## ELECTRICAL THERAPY

Current American Heart Association recommendations for the unstable patient in monomorphic VT are 100, 200, 300, and 360 joules.

## ELECTRICAL THERAPY

Current American Heart Association recommendations for the management of the unstable patient with atrial flutter are:
- synchronized countershock with 50-100-200-300-360 joules.

## ELECTRICAL THERAPY

Assuming the initial quick-look was performed in the paddles simulating electrode positioning for Lead II, rotate the paddles 90 degrees to simulate electrode placement for Lead I or Lead III.

## ELECTRICAL THERAPY

Complications of transcutaneous pacing include:
- Coughing
- Skin burns
- Inability to capture
- Sharp pain or burning sensation with pacing
- Interference with sensing due to muscle contractions or patient agitation.

## ELECTRICAL THERAPY

Current American Heart Association recommendations for the management of the unstable patient with atrial fibrillation are:
- synchronized countershock with 100-200-300-360 joules.

## ELECTRICAL THERAPY

Factors that affect transthoracic resistance include:
- Electrode (paddle) size
- Electrode (paddle) pressure
- Phase of patient's ventilation
- Interelectrode (paddle) distance
- Number and time interval of previous shocks
- Use of interface (gel applied to paddles, use of disposable pads).

## ELECTRICAL THERAPY

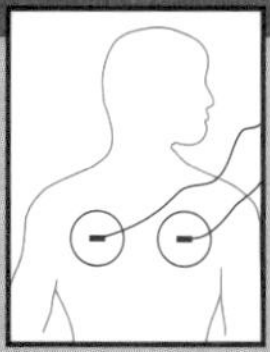

What is the rationale for the delivery of the initial sequence of three "stacked" shocks in ventricular fibrillation or pulseless ventricular tachycardia?

## ELECTRICAL THERAPY

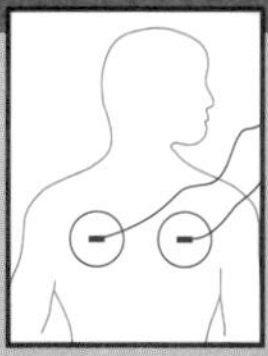

An 80 year old male has suffered a cardiac arrest. The cardiac monitor displays ventricular fibrillation. You have exposed the patient's chest and are preparing to defibrillate when you note the patient has a permanent pacemaker in place.

What distance from the pacemaker generator should the defibrillator paddles be placed?

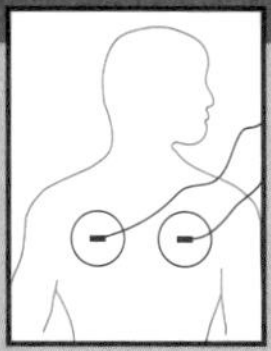

- A 53 year old female is complaining of chest pain and begins losing consciousness. Her BP is now 50/P, respirations 12. The cardiac monitor displays a narrow-QRS tachycardia at 220 beats/minute. Oxygen therapy was initiated and an IV was established prior to the patient's collapse.
- You promptly deliver a synchronized countershock at 50 joules however reassessment reveals the patient to be pulseless and apneic. The cardiac monitor reveals VF.
- What course of action should you take at this time?

## ELECTRICAL THERAPY

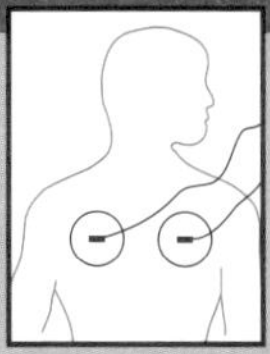

Name three indications for emergent transcutaneous pacing.

## ELECTRICAL THERAPY

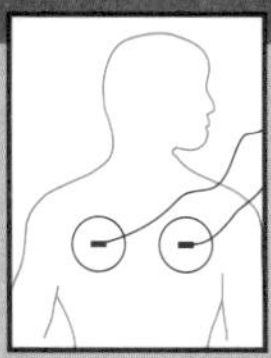

Name four types of vagal maneuvers.

## ELECTRICAL THERAPY

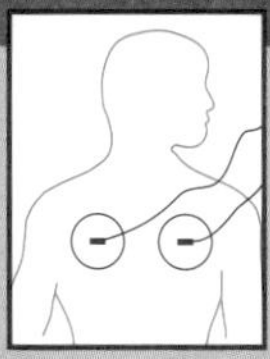

What is the purpose of a vagal maneuver?

## ELECTRICAL THERAPY

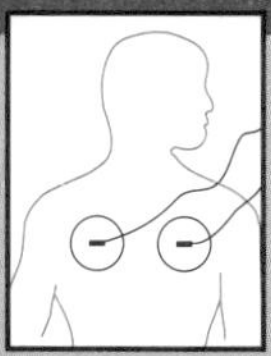

Where is the pulse generator of an automatic implantable-cardioverter defibrillator implanted?

## ELECTRICAL THERAPY

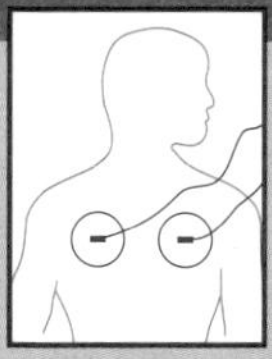

Explain the difference between the AICD and the newer PCD device.

## ELECTRICAL THERAPY

The defibrillator paddles should be placed at least 5 inches (12.5 cm) from the pacemaker generator.

## ELECTRICAL THERAPY

- Defibrillation is the single most important intervention in adult emergency cardiac care.
  - The majority of successful adult resuscitations depend on early defibrillation.
  - The probability of successful defibrillation diminishes rapidly over time.
- Successive shocks are more important that adjunctive drug therapy and delays between shocks to deliver medications are detrimental.
- VF tends to convert to asystole within a few minutes.

## ELECTRICAL THERAPY

- Hemodynamically compromising bradycardias
  - BP < 80 mm Hg systolic, change in mental status, myocardial ischemia, pulmonary edema
- Bradycardia with malignant escape rhythms
  - unresponsive to pharmacologic therapy
- Overdrive pacing of refractory tachycardia
  - SVT or VT refractory to pharmacologic therapy or countershock
- Asystolic cardiac arrest

## ELECTRICAL THERAPY

- Assure the synchronizer switch is off.
- Immediately defibrillate with 200 joules.
- Reassess.

## ELECTRICAL THERAPY

Vagal maneuvers increase parasympathetic tone, thus slowing conduction through the AV node.

## ELECTRICAL THERAPY

Examples of vagal maneuvers:
- coughing
- breath holding
- eyeball pressure
- carotid sinus pressure
- bearing down (Valsalva)
- stimulation of the gag reflex
- facial immersion in ice water

## ELECTRICAL THERAPY

- The AICD (automatic implantable cardioverter-defibrillator) is able to cardiovert VT or defibrillate VF.
- The PCD is an implantable pacer-cardioverter-defibrillator that is designed to deliver tiered therapy. This device:
  - first seeks to correct VT with pacing
  - if overdrive pacing is ineffective, the device will proceed to low-energy cardioversion and, if ineffective, to high-energy cardioversion.
  - The device also provides automatic, programmable ventricular pacing that may be needed in cases of ventricular asystole, intermittent ventricular conduction or post-shock bradycardia.

## ELECTRICAL THERAPY

The pulse generator of the automatic implantable-cardioverter defibrillator (AICD) is implanted in the left upper quadrant of the abdomen.
- The generator consists of a power source capable of shocking the patient approximately 150-200 times, depending on the joule setting and the frequency of shocks.

## ELECTRICAL THERAPY

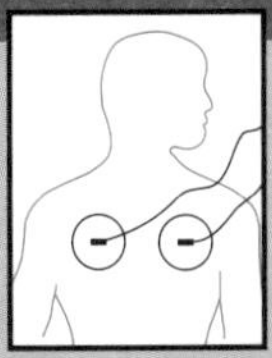

Describe how carotid sinus pressure is performed.

## ELECTRICAL THERAPY

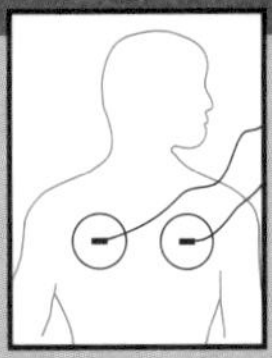

A 78 year old female has suffered a cardiac arrest. The cardiac monitor displays ventricular fibrillation.

As you prepare to defibrillate, where should the defibrillator paddles be placed?

## ELECTRICAL THERAPY

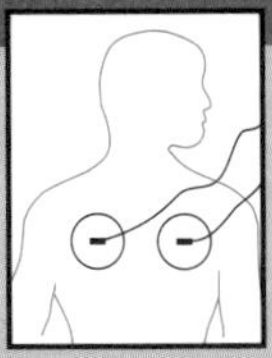

Describe the technique for performing a precordial thump.

## ELECTRICAL THERAPY

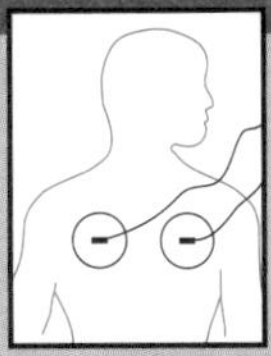

Describe the procedure for performing a "quick-look."

## ELECTRICAL THERAPY

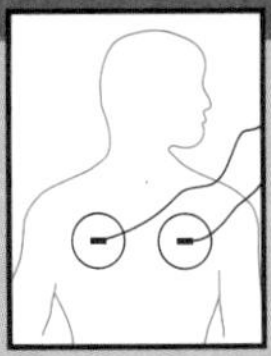

A patient is in cardiac arrest and the quick-look paddles reveal ventricular fibrillation. You note you have inadvertently placed your defibrillator paddles incorrectly (the "apex" paddle has been placed to the right of the sternum and the "sternum" paddle has been placed in the left mid-axillary line).

If you defibrillate with the paddles in their present position, will effectiveness of the defibrillation attempt be affected?

## ELECTRICAL THERAPY

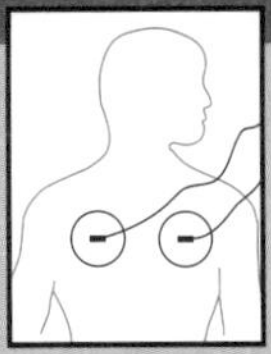

What is meant by the term "cardioversion?"

## ELECTRICAL THERAPY

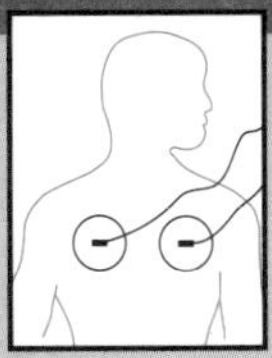

Even properly performed carotid sinus pressure may result in complications.

Name two possible complications of this procedure.

## ELECTRICAL THERAPY

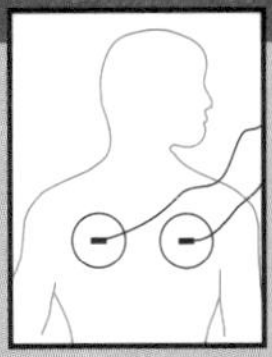

What is the purpose of defibrillation?

## ELECTRICAL THERAPY

- Place the "sternum" paddle to the right of the upper sternum, just below the clavicle.
- Place the "apex" paddle just to the left of the nipple in the mid-axillary line.
  - Anterior-posterior paddle placement may also be used:
    - One paddle is placed to the left of the lower sternal border.
    - The other is positioned on the back behind the heart below the left scapula.

## ELECTRICAL THERAPY

- Carotid sinus pressure should be performed while monitoring the ECG and an IV line, atropine and lidocaine immediately available.
- Turn the patient's head to the left and apply firm momentary pressure on the right carotid bifurcation near the angle of the jaw.
- If unsuccessful, the procedure may be repeated with a "massaging" motion lasting 5-10 seconds.

## ELECTRICAL THERAPY

- Apply gel to the defibrillator paddles or place defib pads on the patient's chest.
- Turn the lead selector on the monitor/defibrillator to "paddles" and turn the power to the machine on.
- Apply the paddles to the patient's chest.
- The paddles will function as electrodes, monitoring the patient's cardiac rhythm while in contact with the patient's chest.

## ELECTRICAL THERAPY

- A precordial thump is delivered to the center of the sternum with the hypothenar aspect of the fist from a height of no more than 12 inches.
- Reassess the rhythm and pulse.
- This procedure is contraindicated in children.

## ELECTRICAL THERAPY

- Some time ago, use of the term "cardioversion" implied the delivery of synchronized countershock.
- Today, this word is used as a general term referring simply to the delivery of energy.
- Specify the TYPE of shock that is to be delivered (synchronized vs unsynchronized countershock).

## ELECTRICAL THERAPY

No, the effectiveness of the defibrillation attempt will not be affected by improper positioning of the sternum and apex paddles.

- The paddle marked "sternum" is the negative electrode and the "apex" paddle is the positive electrode.
- If you placed the quick-look paddles in proper position and viewed a sinus rhythm and then reversed the position of the paddles, you would see a change in the configuration of the P waves on the ECG screen (the P waves would be inverted, indicating a junctional rhythm).
- Although delivery of energy through improperly positioned paddles is not affected, MONITORING of patient (when using defibrillator paddles in quick-look mode) may result in errors in rhythm identification.

## ELECTRICAL THERAPY

The purpose of defibrillation (unsynchronized countershock) is to produce momentary asystole.

- The shock attempts to completely depolarize the myocardium at once and provide an opportunity for the natural pacemaker centers of the heart to resume normal activity.

## ELECTRICAL THERAPY

Possible complications of carotid sinus pressure include:

- Bradycardia
  - AV blocks
  - Asystole
- Ventricular dysrhythmias
- Syncope, seizures or CVA as a result of interference with cerebral circulation.

## ELECTRICAL THERAPY

Why is routine shocking of asystole not recommended?

## ELECTRICAL THERAPY

Management of unstable patients may necessitate the use of electrical therapy.

Identify the correct energy settings for management of an unstable patient with paroxysmal supraventricular tachycardia (PSVT).

## ELECTRICAL THERAPY

Name three contraindications for transcutaneous pacing.

## ELECTRICAL THERAPY

Name three advantages of transcutaneous cardiac pacing.

## ELECTRICAL THERAPY

How does defibrillation differ from synchronized countershock?

## ELECTRICAL THERAPY

Explain the difference between the fully automated and the semi-automated external defibrillator.

## ELECTRICAL THERAPY

What is an AED?

## ELECTRICAL THERAPY

Explain why it is important to look for and remove, if present, transdermal delivery patches from the patient's chest before delivering a countershock.

## ELECTRICAL THERAPY

Current American Heart Association recommendations for the management of the unstable patient with paroxysmal supraventricular tachycardia (PSVT) are:

- synchronized countershock with 50-100-200-300-360 joules.

## ELECTRICAL THERAPY

- Electric shocks produces sympathetic discharge.
- Shocking asystole could eliminate any possibility for return of spontaneous cardiac activity.

## ELECTRICAL THERAPY

Advantages of transcutaneous cardiac pacing include:

- safety
- ease of application
- lack of significant pain
- least invasive pacing technique available
- can be used effectively by prehospital personnel, nurses and other non-physician providers with appropriate training.

## ELECTRICAL THERAPY

Contraindications for transcutaneous pacing include:

- Flail chest
- Chest trauma
- Cervical spine injury
- Weight < 15 kg (33 lbs) unless special pediatric pacing pads are available.

## ELECTRICAL THERAPY

Fully automated defibrillator:

- Requires that the defibrillator pads be attached to the patient and the machine turned on.
- The machine analyzes the rhythm. If VF (or VT above a preset rate) is present, the machine charges its capacitors and delivers a shock.

Semi-automated defibrillator:

- Requires the operator to press an "analyze" control to initiate rhythm analysis and press a "shock" control to deliver the shock.
- The shock control is pressed only when the device identifies VF (or VT above a preset rate) and "advises" the operator to press the shock control.
- Never enters the analysis mode unless activated by the operator.
- Leaves the final decision to shock to the operator.

## ELECTRICAL THERAPY

- Defibrillation (unsynchronized countershock) has no relation to the cardiac cycle (a random discharge of energy).
- Synchronized countershock reduces the potential for delivery of energy during the vulnerable period of the T wave (relative refractory period).
  - A synchronizing circuit searches for the peak of the QRS complex (R wave deflection) and delivers the shock a few milliseconds after the highest part of the R wave.

## ELECTRICAL THERAPY

The aluminized backing used on some transdermal delivery systems can lead to electric arcing during defibrillation with:

- explosive noises
- smoke
- visible arcing
- patient burns
- impaired delivery of current.

## ELECTRICAL THERAPY

- AED = Automated External Defibrillator
- The AED is an external defibrillator with a cardiac rhythm analysis system which senses and records the rhythm and, if indicated, delivers an electrical shock.
  - The shock is delivered by means of two adhesive pads applied to the patient.

## ELECTRICAL THERAPY

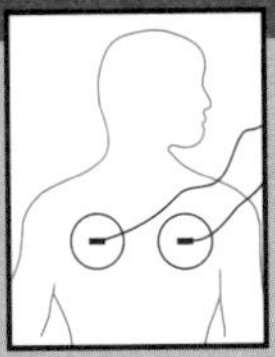

A 75 year old male has suffered a cardiac arrest. The monitor shows ventricular fibrillation.

After you deliver the first shock to this patient, should CPR be resumed while recharging the defibrillator in preparation for the second shock?

## ELECTRICAL THERAPY

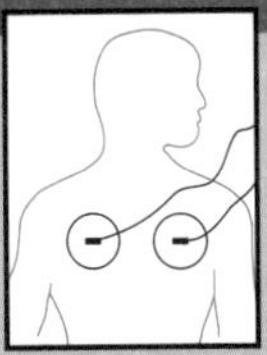

Name two advantages of the automated external defibrillator (AED).

## ELECTRICAL THERAPY

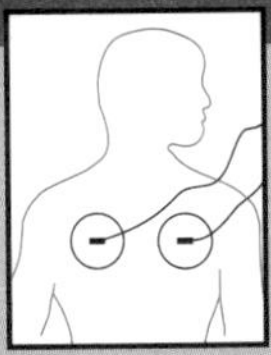

If defibrillation is necessary when transcutaneous pacing electrodes have been applied to the chest, where should the defibrillator paddles be placed?

## ELECTRICAL THERAPY

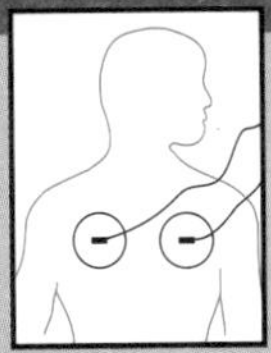

- A 60 year old male arrives in the Emergency Department complaining of chest pain which has been present for 3 hours.
- Administration of oxygen and nitroglycerin has resulted in relief of pain. His blood pressure is now 100/70, pulse rate of 44, respiratory rate 14. The cardiac monitor reveals a second-degree AV block, type II. The 12-lead ECG reveals evidence of an anterior MI.
- What should be done now?

## ELECTRICAL THERAPY

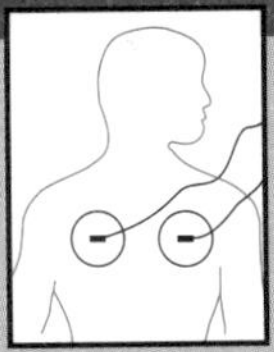

- Basic EMTs responded to a 73 year old male in cardiac arrest. The patient was confirmed to be pulseless and apneic and an automated external defibrillator (AED) was applied. The AED delivered 3 sequential shocks without conversion of the rhythm.
- The patient has now arrived in the Emergency Department. The AED has delivered a second set of 3 sequential shocks without conversion of the rhythm. CPR has been resumed.
- As an ACLS rescuer, how should you proceed?

## ELECTRICAL THERAPY

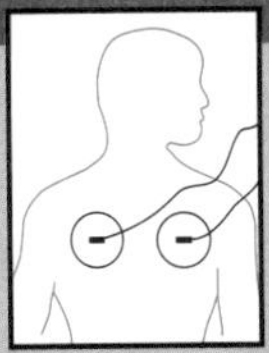

- A 43 year old male is brought to your Emergency Department by Paramedics. The patient is complaining of dizziness and palpitations. Oxygen therapy has been initiated and an IV line is in place.
- The patient has a history of "heart problems" for which he takes Procan SR. His blood pressure is 100/70, respiratory rate 18.
- The cardiac monitor reveals Torsades de Pointes.
- What would you recommend at this point?

## ELECTRICAL THERAPY

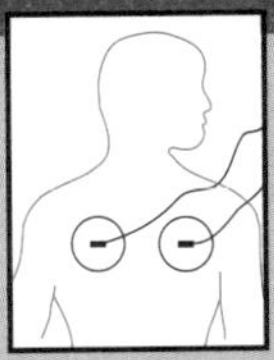

When is the use of an automatic implantable cardioverter-defibrillator (AICD) indicated?

## ELECTRICAL THERAPY

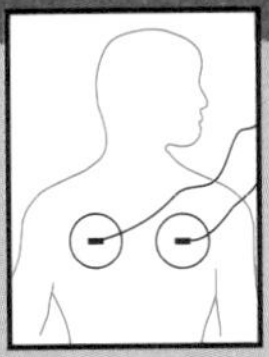

Name two disadvantages of the automated external defibrillator (AED).

## ELECTRICAL THERAPY

- Easy to use
- Reliable performance
- Permits remote, "hands-free" defibrillation
- Less training required to operate and maintain skills
- Speed of operation (delivery of first shock) faster than that with conventional defibrillators

## ELECTRICAL THERAPY

No. Personnel should not perform CPR while the rhythm is reassessed and the defibrillator is recharged.

## ELECTRICAL THERAPY

- Prepare for insertion of a transvenous pacemaker.
- Second-degree AV block, type II may progress rapidly to complete (third-degree AV block) without warning.

## ELECTRICAL THERAPY

If defibrillation is necessary when pacing electrodes have been applied to the chest, the disposable defib pads and paddles should be placed 2-3 cm from the pacemaker electrodes to prevent arcing.

## ELECTRICAL THERAPY

- Discontinue the Procan SR!
- Obtain a 12-lead ECG and draw lab studies to include potassium and magnesium levels.
- Administer magnesium sulfate 1-2 grams IV over 1-2 minutes. Additional magnesium may be administered as needed (repeat bolus therapy or continuous IV infusion).
- Overdrive pacing may be needed if there is no response to treatment with magnesium sulfate.
- If the episodes of torsades are sustained, it may be necessary to perform unsynchronized countershock (200, 200-300, 360J).

## ELECTRICAL THERAPY

- Begin the ACLS ventricular fibrillation sequence - i.e., continue CPR, intubate at once, establish IV access, administered epinephrine, etc.
- ACLS providers should not remove the AED and attach a separate defibrillator unless the AED does not have a rhythm display screen.

## ELECTRICAL THERAPY

- Current AEDs use a liquid crystal display screen that may be less suitable than the bright cathode ray displays of conventional defibrillators.
- The lowest energy setting for currently available AEDs is 200 joules which is high for patients weighing less than 50 kg (110 pounds).
- The AED is not recommended for use with children.

## ELECTRICAL THERAPY

The AICD is indicated for treatment of patients suffering from or at risk for sudden cardiac arrest.

- Candidates for an AICD will have survived at least one episode of cardiac arrest from either VT or VF, not associated with an acute MI

OR

- Have recurrent VT that does not respond to conventional antidysrhythmic drug therapy.

## IV TECHNIQUES

Name four local complications of intravenous therapy.

## IV TECHNIQUES

How would you determine if an IV solution had infiltrated?

## IV TECHNIQUES

A 75 year old male has suffered a cardiac arrest. No IV line is in place.

As the team leader of this resuscitation effort, indicate your sites of first choice in the placement of an IV line in this situation.

## IV TECHNIQUES

Of the following, which is considered a peripheral vein?

- Femoral
- Subclavian
- External jugular
- Internal jugular

## IV TECHNIQUES

What are the preferred IV solutions for use in cardiac arrest?

## IV TECHNIQUES

Name four systemic complications of intravenous therapy.

## IV TECHNIQUES

Name three possible systemic complications of internal jugular or subclavian venipuncture.

## IV TECHNIQUES

Where is the external jugular vein located?

## IV TECHNIQUES

- One of the most reliable methods of evaluating infiltration is to apply a tourniquet above (proximal to) the infusion site tight enough to restrict venous flow. Infiltration is present if the IV solution continues to infuse despite the presence of the venous constricting band.
- Backflow of blood into the IV tubing is not a reliable sign of patency of the IV line. The IV solution will seep into the tissues as well as flow into the vein if the catheter tip has punctured the wall of the vein.
- Other signs of infiltration include pain, pallor, and/or swelling of the IV site, a significant decrease in the infusion rate, coolness in the area of infiltration, or tissue sloughing.

## IV TECHNIQUES

- Phlebitis
- Cellulitis
- Thrombosis
- Hematoma formation
- Infiltration/extravasation

## IV TECHNIQUES

- The external jugular is considered a peripheral vein.
- The internal jugular, subclavian and femoral veins are central veins.

## IV TECHNIQUES

If no IV exists at the time of the arrest, sites of first choice are the antecubital or external jugular veins.

## IV TECHNIQUES

- Sepsis
- Air embolism
- Circulatory overload
- Catheter-fragment embolism
- Pulmonary thromboembolism

## IV TECHNIQUES

- The preferred IV solutions in cardiac arrest are normal saline and lactated Ringer's
- 5% dextrose in water is acceptable, but not preferred.

## IV TECHNIQUES

- The external jugular vein lies superficially along the lateral portion of the neck.
- It extends from the angle of the mandible and passes downward until it enters the thorax at a point just above the middle of the clavicle and ends in the subclavian vein.

## IV TECHNIQUES

- Hemothorax
- Air embolism
- Pneumothorax
- Dysrhythmias from the catheter tip
- Infiltration into the mediastinum or pleural space

## IV TECHNIQUES

Name three advantages of peripheral venipuncture.

## IV TECHNIQUES

Why is the intramuscular medication route generally avoided in cardiac arrest?

## IV TECHNIQUES

Name three indications for central venous access.

## IV TECHNIQUES

Name three disadvantages of subclavian venipuncture.

## IV TECHNIQUES

Name two advantages of femoral vein cannulation.

## IV TECHNIQUES

Name a possible complication associated with the use of a catheter-through-the-needle device.

## IV TECHNIQUES

Name three advantages of internal jugular vein cannulation.

## IV TECHNIQUES

Name two indications for intravenous cannulation.

## IV TECHNIQUES

Intramuscular injections cause a release of creatine phosphokinase (CPK) from the local area of muscle into the central circulation, altering the diagnostic usefulness of this enzyme in indicating myocardial necrosis.

## IV TECHNIQUES

- Easy to learn.
- Does not require interruption of CPR.
- Is an effective route for medication administration.
- Results in fewer complications than central venous access.

## IV TECHNIQUES

- May interrupt CPR
- More training required than with peripheral venipuncture
- Higher complication rate than with peripheral venipuncture
- Significant risk of pneumothorax, hemothorax and/or subclavian artery puncture
- Increased risk of complications associated with central line placement for patients who receive thrombolytic therapy.

## IV TECHNIQUES

- Central venous pressure measurement
- Emergency access to venous circulation
- Administration of hypertonic or irritating solutions
- Passing catheters into the heart and pulmonary circulation.

## IV TECHNIQUES

When using a catheter-through-the-needle device, there is a risk of the sharp tip of the needle shearing off the end of the catheter, producing a catheter-fragment embolus.

- Never pull backward through the needle.
- If you cannot advance the catheter through the needle, you must remove both the needle and the catheter.

## IV TECHNIQUES

- Does not interrupt CPR
- Vein does not collapse like peripheral veins
- Once cannulated, there is easy access to the central circulation.

## IV TECHNIQUES

Indications for IV cannulation include:

- to obtain venous blood for laboratory analysis
- to provide a route for medication administration
- to replace water and correct electrolyte deficits
- to insert catheters into the central circulation for physiological monitoring and electrical pacing.

## IV TECHNIQUES

- Easier access during CPR than subclavian approach.
- Less risk of pneumothorax with this technique than subclavian.
- Hematomas in the neck are visible and more easily compressible.
- Rapid access to the central circulation is possible even if peripheral veins are collapsed.

## IV TECHNIQUES

Name two advantages of external jugular vein cannulation.

## IV TECHNIQUES

Why are the intravenous and endotracheal routes preferred over intracardiac injection as a method of medication administration in cardiac arrest?

## IV TECHNIQUES

Name two disadvantages of femoral vein cannulation.

## IV TECHNIQUES

Describe two signs and symptoms of thrombophlebitis.

## IV TECHNIQUES

Name three signs and symptoms of circulatory overload.

## IV TECHNIQUES

Name three disadvantages of peripheral venipuncture.

## IV TECHNIQUES

Why is the right side of the neck preferred when cannulating the internal jugular vein?

## IV TECHNIQUES

Where is the femoral vein relative to the femoral artery?

## IV TECHNIQUES

- Intracardiac injection is associated with significant complications.
- The major hazard associated with intracardiac injection is the need to interrupt CPR to perform the procedure.
- Other complications of intracardiac injection include:
  - pneumothorax, pneumopericardium, myocardial laceration, intramyocardial injection, coronary artery laceration, internal mammary artery laceration, hemopericardium (with or without tamponade).

## IV TECHNIQUES

- Usually easy to cannulate
- Is considered a peripheral vein
- Provides rapid access to the central circulation.

## IV TECHNIQUES

- Heat, pain, redness, and swelling along the affected vessel.
- The affected vein may also appear hard or cord-like.

## IV TECHNIQUES

- If the pulse is absent, the vein may be hard to locate.
- Long delivery time of drugs into the central circulation unless a long line that extends above the diaphragm is used.
  - due to decreased flow to the extremities
- Complication rate (thrombosis, infection) may be higher than for peripheral veins.

## IV TECHNIQUES

- Delay of 1-2 minutes for drugs to reach the central circulation in cardiac arrest.
- It may be difficult or impossible to establish an IV via a peripheral vein in cases of circulatory collapse.
- Pain and phlebitis may result if peripheral veins are used to administer hypertonic or irritating solutions.

## IV TECHNIQUES

- Cough
- Rales
- Chest pain
- Tachycardia
- Pulmonary edema
- Shortness of breath
- Distended neck veins
- Congestive heart failure

## IV TECHNIQUES

The femoral vein lies in the femoral sheath medial to the femoral artery, immediately below the inguinal ligament.

## IV TECHNIQUES

- The thoracic duct is not in the way.
  - the thoracic duct empties on the LEFT side
- There is more or less a straight line to the right atrium.
- The dome of the right lung and pleura are lower than on the left.

## IV TECHNIQUES

What is meant by the term "Seldinger technique"?

## IV TECHNIQUES

Describe how you would manage the patient who suffered an air embolism as a result of IV therapy.

## IV TECHNIQUES

Name two possible complications of femoral venipuncture.

## IV TECHNIQUES

You are attempting to cannulate the femoral vein and note the appearance of bright red blood in the syringe.

How will you manage this situation?

## IV TECHNIQUES

Describe the proper technique for applying a tourniquet prior to intravenous cannulation.

## IV TECHNIQUES

Name two veins of the upper extremity commonly used for intravenous therapy.

## IV TECHNIQUES

- Stop the IV infusion and check for air or leaks in the IV tubing.
- Turn the patient on his/her left side with the head down.
  - This position may facilitate the movement of air to the right side of the heart and help minimize the movement of air into the arterial circulation.
- Administer high flow oxygen.

## IV TECHNIQUES

Seldinger technique refers to insertion of a catheter over a guidewire.

- A venipuncture is made with a needle.
- A guidewire is inserted into the vein through the needle and the needle is removed.
- A catheter is then inserted over the guidewire into the vein and the guidewire is removed.

## IV TECHNIQUES

- The appearance of bright red blood in the syringe indicates cannulation of the femoral artery.
- Withdraw the needle and apply firm pressure to the puncture site for 10 minutes.

## IV TECHNIQUES

Possible complications of femoral venipuncture include:

- Hematoma
- Thrombosis and phlebitis
- Inadvertent cannulation of the femoral artery.

## IV TECHNIQUES

Veins of the upper extremity commonly used for intravenous therapy include:

- the metacarpal veins of the hand
- the radial and ulnar veins of the forearm
- the median basilic and median cephalic veins which form a Y at the antecubital fossa
- the basilic and cephalic veins of the upper arm.

## IV TECHNIQUES

- The tourniquet should be applied tight enough to restrict venous blood flow without cutting off the arterial circulation.
- The tourniquet is too tight if a pulse cannot be palpated below the tourniquet site.

## CARDIOVASCULAR PHARMACOLOGY

What is the usual dosage range for dobutamine administration?

## CARDIOVASCULAR PHARMACOLOGY

Name four indications for lidocaine administration.

## CARDIOVASCULAR PHARMACOLOGY

Name four clinical indications of lidocaine toxicity.

## CARDIOVASCULAR PHARMACOLOGY

Name three side effects associated with the use of nitrates.

## CARDIOVASCULAR PHARMACOLOGY

What is the recommended dose of atropine in the treatment of asystole?

## CARDIOVASCULAR PHARMACOLOGY

When should the dosage of lidocaine be reduced?

## CARDIOVASCULAR PHARMACOLOGY

Name three precautions that should be observed when administering sodium nitroprusside.

## CARDIOVASCULAR PHARMACOLOGY

What is the recommended dosage range for morphine sulfate administration?

## CARDIOVASCULAR PHARMACOLOGY

Lidocaine is recommended in:
- VT with a pulse
- Wide-complex tachycardia of uncertain origin
- Control of significant PVCs in the setting of ischemia/infarction
- Pulseless VT and VF that persist after defibrillation and administration of epinephrine

## CARDIOVASCULAR PHARMACOLOGY

The usual dosage range is 2-20 ug/kg/min.
- Increases in heart rate of more than 10% may induce or exacerbate myocardial ischemia.
- Hemodynamic monitoring is recommended.

## CARDIOVASCULAR PHARMACOLOGY

- Headaches (most common) due to dilation of the cerebral vessels.
- Dizziness
- Flushing
- Nausea/vomiting
- Reflex tachycardia
  - Vasodilation occurs as a result of nitrate administration, pooling blood in the periphery. The decrease in arterial pressure stimulates baroreceptors, resulting in stimulation of the sympathetic division of the autonomic nervous system.

## CARDIOVASCULAR PHARMACOLOGY

Indications of lidocaine toxicity are usually central nervous system related and include:
- Dizziness
- Drowsiness
- Mild agitation
- Hearing impairment
- Disorientation and confusion
- Muscle twitching
- Seizures
- Respiratory arrest

## CARDIOVASCULAR PHARMACOLOGY

- The dose of lidocaine should be reduced in:
  - decreased cardiac output
  - acute MI
  - congestive heart failure
  - shock from any cause
  - patients older than 70 years
  - hepatic dysfunction
- These patients should receive the normal bolus dose, followed by 1/2 the normal maintenance infusion.

## CARDIOVASCULAR PHARMACOLOGY

- The recommended intravenous dose for atropine in the treatment of asystole is 1 mg repeated every 3-5 minutes to a maximum dose of 3 mg (approximately 0.04 mg/kg).
  - The 3 mg dose is thought to result in full vagal blockade.
- The recommended endotracheal dose is 2-2.5 times the IV dose (2-2.5 mg) diluted in 10 ml of normal saline or distilled water.

## CARDIOVASCULAR PHARMACOLOGY

Morphine should be administered in small IV increments (1-3 mg) repeated as often as every 5 minutes if necessary, titrated to desired analgesic or hemodynamic effect, provided the patient's systolic blood pressure remains > 100 and respiratory rate remains adequate.

## CARDIOVASCULAR PHARMACOLOGY

- Protect from light by wrapping the IV bag in the aluminum foil package provided.
- Do not add other medications to this IV solution.
- Should be infused via an infusion pump.
- Sodium nitroprusside normally has a brownish tint when reconstituted. Discard the solution if it is strongly discolored.
- Use the solution within four hours of preparation.
- Watch for symptoms of thiocyanate toxicity (disorientation, metabolic acidosis, nausea, muscle spasms, absent reflexes).

## CARDIOVASCULAR PHARMACOLOGY

List two indications for the use of verapamil.

## CARDIOVASCULAR PHARMACOLOGY

What is the primary neurotransmitter of the parasympathetic division of the autonomic nervous system?

## CARDIOVASCULAR PHARMACOLOGY

Describe the procedure for administration of drugs by means of the endotracheal route in cardiac arrest.

## CARDIOVASCULAR PHARMACOLOGY

When should an infusion of procainamide be discontinued?

## CARDIOVASCULAR PHARMACOLOGY

Describe how to prepare an isoproterenol infusion.

## CARDIOVASCULAR PHARMACOLOGY

Name three indications for bretylium administration.

## CARDIOVASCULAR PHARMACOLOGY

How does bretylium administration differ for the patient in pulseless VT/VF from the patient in VT with a pulse?

## CARDIOVASCULAR PHARMACOLOGY

What is the recommended dosage range for the administration of Verapamil?

## CARDIOVASCULAR PHARMACOLOGY

Acetylcholine is the primary neurotransmitter of the parasympathetic division of the autonomic nervous system.

## CARDIOVASCULAR PHARMACOLOGY

Verapamil is indicated in:

- narrow-complex PSVT (adenosine is the drug of choice)
- atrial fibrillation or atrial flutter with a rapid ventricular response
- wide-complex tachycardia KNOWN WITH CERTAINTY to be supraventricular in origin
  - Administration of verapamil to a patient with VT may be lethal.

## CARDIOVASCULAR PHARMACOLOGY

Procainamide should be discontinued if any of the following occurs:

- Hypotension develops
- The dysrhythmia is suppressed
- The QRS widens by more than 50% of its original width
- A total of 17 mg/kg has been administered
  - (approximately 1.2 grams for a 70 kg patient).

## CARDIOVASCULAR PHARMACOLOGY

- The American Heart Association recommends passing a catheter beyond the tip of the endotracheal tube.
- If the needle and syringe are not a single unit (most preloads are a single unit), remove the needle from the syringe.
- Momentarily stop CPR and disconnect the bag-valve device from the endotracheal tube. Quickly administer the medication down the endotracheal tube.
- Once the medication has been administered, deliver several forceful insufflations of the bag-valve device to enhance drug absorption.
- Resume CPR.

## CARDIOVASCULAR PHARMACOLOGY

Bretylium is indicated:

- After defibrillation, epinephrine and lidocaine have failed to convert VF
- VF has recurred despite epinephrine and lidocaine
- Lidocaine and procainamide have failed to control VT with a pulse
- Lidocaine and adenosine have failed to convert a wide-complex tachycardia.

## CARDIOVASCULAR PHARMACOLOGY

- To prepare an isoproterenol infusion, mix 1 mg of isoproterenol in 250 ml of IV solution (this produces a concentration of 4 mcg/ml)
- Using this concentration and an administration set that delivers 60 gtts/ml:
  - 1 mcg/min = 15 gtts/min
  - 2 mcg/min = 30 gtts/min
  - 3 mcg/min = 45 gtts/min
  - 4 mcg/min = 60 gtts/min

## CARDIOVASCULAR PHARMACOLOGY

- The recommended dosage of Verapamil is 2.5-5.0 mg SLOW IV bolus over 2 minutes.
- If no response to the initial dose (and the patient's blood pressure is normal or elevated), repeat with 5-10 mg every 15-30 minutes to a maximum dose of 20 mg.

## CARDIOVASCULAR PHARMACOLOGY

- In pulseless VT and VF, bretylium is administered as an IV BOLUS.
  - Initial dose 5 mg/kg
  - May be repeated with 10 mg/kg in 5 minutes to a maximum dose of 30-35 mg/kg
- In persistently recurring VT with a pulse, bretylium is diluted in 50 ml of IV solution and infused over 8-10 minutes.

## CARDIOVASCULAR PHARMACOLOGY

When should amrinone (Inocor) be considered?

## CARDIOVASCULAR PHARMACOLOGY

Name two indications for administration of morphine sulfate.

## CARDIOVASCULAR PHARMACOLOGY

Name two indications for administration of an isoproterenol infusion.

## CARDIOVASCULAR PHARMACOLOGY

Name two precautions that should be observed when administering amrinone (Inocor).

## CARDIOVASCULAR PHARMACOLOGY

Describe the effects of dopamine administration at 1-2 mcg/kg/minute.

## CARDIOVASCULAR PHARMACOLOGY

Of the following, which are administered only by continuous intravenous infusion?

- dopamine
- atropine
- isoproterenol
- lidocaine
- dobutamine

## CARDIOVASCULAR PHARMACOLOGY

Compare the cardiovascular effects of diltiazem and verapamil.

## CARDIOVASCULAR PHARMACOLOGY

Explain the mechanism of action of calcium channel blockers.

## CARDIOVASCULAR PHARMACOLOGY

Morphine sulfate is indicated in:
- acute myocardial infarction
- acute pulmonary edema
  - Class IIb (possibly helpful)

## CARDIOVASCULAR PHARMACOLOGY

Amrinone should be considered in patients with severe congestive heart failure refractory to diuretics, vasodilators and conventional inotropic agents.

## CARDIOVASCULAR PHARMACOLOGY

- Amrinone should be clear yellow. The solution should be discarded if it is discolored or if it is more than 24 hours old.
- Amrinone should not be administered in the same IV line as furosemide (Lasix) as these drugs are incompatible.
- Amrinone should be administered via an infusion pump.
- Amrinone should not be diluted with solutions containing dextrose because dextrose inactivates this medication.
- Amrinone can induce or worsen myocardial ischemia. Hemodynamic monitoring is essential for proper dosing.

## CARDIOVASCULAR PHARMACOLOGY

- Isoproterenol is considered Class IIa (probably helpful) for refractory Torsades de Pointes
  - Magnesium sulfate is the drug of choice
- Symptomatic bradycardia (consider after atropine, pacing, dopamine and epinephrine infusion)
  - Class IIb (possibly helpful) at low doses
  - Class III (possibly harmful) at high doses

## CARDIOVASCULAR PHARMACOLOGY

- Dopamine, isoproterenol and dobutamine are administered as continuous IV infusions, not as IV bolus medications.
- Atropine is administered as an IV bolus.
- Lidocaine is administered first as an IV bolus and followed with a continuous IV infusion.

## CARDIOVASCULAR PHARMACOLOGY

At 1-2 mcg/kg/min, dopamine dilates the renal and mesenteric vasculature.

## CARDIOVASCULAR PHARMACOLOGY

- Calcium channel blockers act directly and indirectly on the heart by inhibiting the influx of calcium ions across the cell membrane of cardiac and smooth muscle cells.
- The slow influx of calcium causes these cells to contract more slowly, thereby decreasing contractility and increasing vasodilation.
  - Rosalinda Alfaro-LeFevre et al., *Drug Handbook, A Nursing Process Approach* (Redwood City, CA: Addison-Wesley Nursing, 1992), 44.

## CARDIOVASCULAR PHARMACOLOGY

- Although diltiazem and verapamil are calcium channel blockers, their cardiovascular effects differ.
- Verapamil:
  - more pronounced depressant effect on AV nodal conduction
  - more pronounced negative inotropic effect (decreased myocardial contractility)
- Diltiazem:
  - more pronounced effect on peripheral arterial vasodilation
  - more pronounced depressant effect on the SA node.

## CARDIOVASCULAR PHARMACOLOGY

Name three indications for calcium chloride administration.

## CARDIOVASCULAR PHARMACOLOGY

Name the primary target organs affected by stimulation of the following receptor sites:

- alpha-1
- beta-1
- beta-2

## CARDIOVASCULAR PHARMACOLOGY

Name three objectives of drug therapy in advanced cardiac life support.

## CARDIOVASCULAR PHARMACOLOGY

Define "inotrope."

## CARDIOVASCULAR PHARMACOLOGY

Describe the effects of dopamine administration at an infusion rate of greater than 20 mcg/kg/minute.

## CARDIOVASCULAR PHARMACOLOGY

Name the adrenergic-receptor sites stimulated by epinephrine.

## CARDIOVASCULAR PHARMACOLOGY

Name three side effects of atropine administration.

## CARDIOVASCULAR PHARMACOLOGY

Describe the effects of atropine on the cardiac conduction system.

## CARDIOVASCULAR PHARMACOLOGY

- Alpha-1 receptor sites are located in vascular smooth muscle.
- Beta-1 (one heart) receptor sites are located in the heart.
- Beta-2 (two lungs) receptor sites are located in the smooth muscle of the bronchi and skeletal blood vessels.

## CARDIOVASCULAR PHARMACOLOGY

Calcium chloride is considered a Class IIa (probably helpful) intervention in:

- hyperkalemia
- hypocalcemia
- calcium channel blocker toxicity/overdose

## CARDIOVASCULAR PHARMACOLOGY

Inotrope refers to myocardial contractility.

- A positive inotropic effect refers to an increase in myocardial contractility.
- A negative inotropic effect refers to a decrease in myocardial contractility.

## CARDIOVASCULAR PHARMACOLOGY

Objectives of drug therapy in Advanced Cardiac Life Support include:

- to relieve pain
- to correct acidosis
- to correct hypoxemia
- to optimize cardiac function
- to treat congestive heart failure
- to reestablish spontaneous circulation
- to suppress sustained ventricular dysrhythmias.

## CARDIOVASCULAR PHARMACOLOGY

Epinephrine stimulates alpha and beta-adrenergic receptor sites.

## CARDIOVASCULAR PHARMACOLOGY

- At an infusion rate of greater than 20 mcg/kg/minute, dopamine's effects are purely alpha resulting in:
  - renal and mesenteric vasoconstriction
  - peripheral arterial and venous vasoconstriction
- Effects at this dosage are similar to those of norepinephrine

## CARDIOVASCULAR PHARMACOLOGY

Atropine competes with acetylcholine at receptor sites, blocking the parasympathetic response (vagolytic action). As a result, administration of atropine should result in:

- acceleration of the rate of discharge of the SA node
  - by increasing the sinus rate, atropine may decrease the incidence of ectopic ventricular activity.
- improved AV conduction.

## CARDIOVASCULAR PHARMACOLOGY

- Cardiovascular:
  - Palpitations, tachycardia, possible extension of MI, angina, ventricular ectopy
- CNS:
  - Anxiety, dizziness, headache, confusion, delirium
- Other:
  - Blurred vision, pupil dilation
  - Dry mouth, acute urine retention
  - Decreased sweating, flushed skin

## CARDIOVASCULAR PHARMACOLOGY

Of the following, which are ventricular antidysrhythmic agents?

- Lidocaine
- Bretylium
- Verapamil
- Dopamine
- Procainamide

## CARDIOVASCULAR PHARMACOLOGY

Name three medications that may be administered via the endotracheal route in the adult patient.

## CARDIOVASCULAR PHARMACOLOGY

Name six absolute contraindications for thrombolytic therapy.

## CARDIOVASCULAR PHARMACOLOGY

Name three indications for administration of magnesium sulfate.

## CARDIOVASCULAR PHARMACOLOGY

What is the usual dosage of Lasix?

How might the initial dose of this drug be adjusted if a patient is already taking the drug orally?

## CARDIOVASCULAR PHARMACOLOGY

Which of the following exert a positive dromotropic action?

- digitalis
- verapamil
- epinephrine
- norepinephrine

## CARDIOVASCULAR PHARMACOLOGY

- Resuscitation efforts are in progress for a 64 year old female in VF. CPR is being properly performed. Administration of epinephrine and a total of 3 mg/kg of lidocaine have proven unsuccessful. You instruct a team member to administer a 5 mg/kg bolus of bretylium and defibrillate with 360J within 30-60 seconds.
- After administration of bretylium and defibrillation, the cardiac monitor displays a sinus rhythm at 80 beats/minute. A weak pulse is present. BP is 96/60. There are no spontaneous respirations.
- What should be done now?

## CARDIOVASCULAR PHARMACOLOGY

Name three indications for procainamide administration.

## CARDIOVASCULAR PHARMACOLOGY

The following medications may be administered via the endotracheal route in the adult patient and may be remembered by the use of LEAN, LANE or NEAL:

- Lidocaine
- Atropine
- Naloxone (Narcan)
- Epinephrine

## CARDIOVASCULAR PHARMACOLOGY

- Ventricular antidysrhythmics include:
    - Lidocaine
    - Bretylium
    - Procainamide
- Verapamil is a calcium channel blocker used in the treatment of PSVT, atrial fibrillation and atrial flutter with a rapid ventricular response.
- Dopamine is a vasopressor used in the treatment of hemodynamically significant hypotension (in the absence of hypovolemia).

## CARDIOVASCULAR PHARMACOLOGY

Magnesium sulfate is indicated in:

- Pulseless VT/VF
- Hypomagnesemia
- Torsades de Pointes
- Acute myocardial infarction

## CARDIOVASCULAR PHARMACOLOGY

- Pregnancy
- Active internal bleeding
- Suspected aortic aneurysm or acute pericarditis
- Prolonged and/or traumatic CPR (>5-10 minutes)
- Recent head trauma or known intracranial neoplasm
- Severe trauma or major surgery (within past 2 weeks)
- History of recent CVA or TIA (within previous 6 months)
- Previous allergic reaction to the thrombolytic agent being considered
- Severe persistent hypertension (>180 mm Hg systolic or >110 mm Hg diastolic) not readily responsive to pain relief or initial pharmacologic measures.

## CARDIOVASCULAR PHARMACOLOGY

- Epinephrine and norepinephrine speed conduction through the AV node (positive dromotropic effect).
- Digitalis and verapamil slow or delay conduction through the AV node (negative dromotropic effect).

## CARDIOVASCULAR PHARMACOLOGY

- The usual dose of lasix (furosemide) is 0.5-1.0 mg/kg IV bolus.
- If a patient is already taking the medication orally, the physician may choose to order an initial dose of lasix that is twice the daily oral dose.

## CARDIOVASCULAR PHARMACOLOGY

Procainamide is recommended when lidocaine is contraindicated or has failed to suppress ventricular ectopy.

- Refractory pulseless VT/VF
- Suppression of recurrent VT that cannot be controlled with lidocaine
- Atrial fibrillation with a rapid ventricular response (not a first-line drug)
- Wide-complex tachycardia that cannot be distinguished from VT (not a first-line drug).

## CARDIOVASCULAR PHARMACOLOGY

- Continue ventilating the patient and frequently reassess vital signs.
- Since bretylium was the last antidysrhythmic administered, prepare a continuous bretylium infusion and infuse at a rate of 1-2 mg/minute.

## CARDIOVASCULAR PHARMACOLOGY

Define "chronotrope."

## CARDIOVASCULAR PHARMACOLOGY

Name three possible actions/effects of magnesium sulfate.

## CARDIOVASCULAR PHARMACOLOGY

What is the usual dose of calcium chloride?

## CARDIOVASCULAR PHARMACOLOGY

How is adenosine administered?

## CARDIOVASCULAR PHARMACOLOGY

You are instructed to administer a dobutamine infusion at a rate of 5 mcg/kg/minute.

Name two effects of dobutamine when administered at this rate.

## CARDIOVASCULAR PHARMACOLOGY

Describe the effects of digitalis on heart rate and myocardial contractility.

## CARDIOVASCULAR PHARMACOLOGY

Does administration of verapamil affect myocardial contractility?

## CARDIOVASCULAR PHARMACOLOGY

Name three signs/symptoms of magnesium overdose.

## CARDIOVASCULAR PHARMACOLOGY

Magnesium sulfate may decrease the incidence of early MI mortality due to:
- coronary vasodilation
- decreased platelet aggregation
- improved myocardial metabolism
- decreased myocardial infarct size
- protection against catecholamine induced myocardial necrosis
- systemic vasodilation, thus decreasing myocardial oxygen demand.

## CARDIOVASCULAR PHARMACOLOGY

Chronotrope refers to heart rate.
- A positive chronotropic effect refers to an increase in heart rate.
- A negative chronotropic effect refers to a decrease in heart rate.

## CARDIOVASCULAR PHARMACOLOGY

- Due to its extremely short half-life, adenosine should be administered via a large-bore IV line initiated as close to the heart as possible (such as the antecubital vein).
- The initial bolus is 6 mg RAPID IV bolus over 1-3 seconds followed by a 20 ml saline flush and elevation of the extremity. If no response, may repeat with 12 mg in 1-2 min. The 12 mg dose may be repeated once in 1-2 minutes.

## CARDIOVASCULAR PHARMACOLOGY

- The dose of calcium chloride is 2-4 mg/kg (usually 500 mg-1 gram) of 10% solution.
- Calcium should be administered SLOWLY IV bolus.

## CARDIOVASCULAR PHARMACOLOGY

Digitalis:
- slows heart rate (negative chronotrope)
- increases myocardial contractility (positive inotrope).

## CARDIOVASCULAR PHARMACOLOGY

Dobutamine is a pure beta-adrenergic stimulator, thus effects at 5 mcg/kg/min may result in:
- increased myocardial contractility
  - potent INOTROPIC agent
- increased cardiac output
  - increased myocardial contractility - increased stroke volume - increased cardiac output
- increased myocardial oxygen requirements.

## CARDIOVASCULAR PHARMACOLOGY

Signs and symptoms of magnesium overdose include:
- hypotension
- flushing, sweating
- bradycardia, AV block
- respiratory depression
- drowsiness, decreasing level of consciousness
- diminished reflexes or muscle weakness, flaccid paralysis.

## CARDIOVASCULAR PHARMACOLOGY

- Yes. Verapamil is a calcium channel blocker and is a negative inotrope (decreases the force of myocardial contraction).
- Verapamil should be avoided or used with caution in patients with left ventricular dysfunction.

## CARDIOVASCULAR PHARMACOLOGY

Describe the mechanism of action of sodium nitroprusside.

## CARDIOVASCULAR PHARMACOLOGY

What is the usual dose of norepinephrine?

## CARDIOVASCULAR PHARMACOLOGY

When is administration of norepinephrine indicated?

## CARDIOVASCULAR PHARMACOLOGY

What is the initial and repeat dosing schedule for sodium bicarbonate administration?

## CARDIOVASCULAR PHARMACOLOGY

When is sodium bicarbonate administration considered a Class I (definitely helpful) intervention?

## CARDIOVASCULAR PHARMACOLOGY

How is magnesium sulfate administered to the patient in Torsades de Pointes?

## CARDIOVASCULAR PHARMACOLOGY

Relaxation of the bronchi and vasodilation are effects that may be seen with stimulation of __ receptor sites.

## CARDIOVASCULAR PHARMACOLOGY

Describe the effects of dopamine administration at an infusion rate of 2-10 mcg/kg/minute.

## CARDIOVASCULAR PHARMACOLOGY

- The usual dose of norepinephrine is 0.5-30 mcg/minute, titrated to effect.
- Norepinephrine is administered as a continuous infusion that may be prepared by mixing 4 mg of norepinephrine in 250 ml of IV solution.
  - This produces a concentration of 16 mcg/ml.

## CARDIOVASCULAR PHARMACOLOGY

Sodium nitroprusside (Nipride) is a potent, rapid-acting peripheral vasodilator (arterial and venous):
- increases cardiac output
- decreases preload and afterload
- decreases myocardial oxygen requirements.

## CARDIOVASCULAR PHARMACOLOGY

- The initial dose of sodium bicarbonate is 1 mEq/kg.
- The repeat dose is 1/2 the initial dose every 10 minutes thereafter.

## CARDIOVASCULAR PHARMACOLOGY

Norepinephrine (Levophed) is indicated in:
- cardiogenic shock
- severe hypotension (systolic BP < 70 mm Hg)

## CARDIOVASCULAR PHARMACOLOGY

- Administer 1-2 grams IV bolus (2-4 ml of a 50% solution) diluted in 10 ml over 2 minutes. This is often followed with the same amount mixed in 50-100 ml of IV solution over 1 hour.
- Magnesium sulfate is supplied in many dilutions. One such dilution is 1 gram in 2 ml. To administer a 2 gram IV bolus, draw up a total of 4 ml (2 of the 1 gram/2 ml) and dilute with 6 ml of normal saline.

## CARDIOVASCULAR PHARMACOLOGY

Sodium bicarbonate administration is considered a Class I (definitely helpful) intervention in known pre-existing hyperkalemia.

## CARDIOVASCULAR PHARMACOLOGY

At 2-10 mcg/kg/minute, dopamine predominately stimulates beta-adrenergic receptor sites which should result in:
- increased heart rate
- increased force of contraction
- increased cardiac output

## CARDIOVASCULAR PHARMACOLOGY

Stimulation of beta-2 receptor sites results in relaxation of the smooth muscle of the bronchi and peripheral vasodilation.

## CARDIOVASCULAR PHARMACOLOGY

Name the drug that should be on hand for IV administration if signs of overdose develop during administration of magnesium sulfate.

## CARDIOVASCULAR PHARMACOLOGY

Name three indications for oxygen administration.

## CARDIOVASCULAR PHARMACOLOGY

Describe the primary beneficial effects of epinephrine administration in cardiac arrest.

## CARDIOVASCULAR PHARMACOLOGY

Name two complications associated with sodium bicarbonate therapy in cardiac arrest.

## CARDIOVASCULAR PHARMACOLOGY

What is the dose of epinephrine when administered endotracheally?

## CARDIOVASCULAR PHARMACOLOGY

A 50 year old female suddenly develops a rapid heart rate. The cardiac monitor displays a narrow-QRS tachycardia at 180 beats/minute. The patient is awake, alert and denies chest pain or difficulty breathing. Her blood pressure is 128/74.

Name three medications that may be ordered to slow her heart rate.

## CARDIOVASCULAR PHARMACOLOGY

Name two indications for diltiazem administration.

## CARDIOVASCULAR PHARMACOLOGY

Stimulation of beta-adrenergic receptor sites should result in improved myocardial contractility and increased heart rate

Why aren't pure beta-adrenergic stimulating agents (such as isoproterenol) used in the management of cardiac arrest?

## CARDIOVASCULAR PHARMACOLOGY

- Ischemic chest pain
- Cardiac or pulmonary arrest
- Suspected hypoxemia of any cause

## CARDIOVASCULAR PHARMACOLOGY

Calcium chloride.

## CARDIOVASCULAR PHARMACOLOGY

Complications associated with sodium bicarbonate therapy in cardiac arrest include:

- Alkalosis
- Hypernatremia
- Hyperosmolarity
- Shift in the oxyhemoglobin dissociation curve
- Paradoxical intracellular acidosis
    - due to a more rapid diffusion of $CO_2$ into the cells than bicarbonate

## CARDIOVASCULAR PHARMACOLOGY

- Epinephrine stimulates alpha and beta-adrenergic receptor sites.
- The primary beneficial effect of epinephrine administration in cardiac arrest is due to its alpha-adrenergic receptor stimulating action, resulting in peripheral vasoconstriction.
    - Increased peripheral vasoconstriction improves cerebral and coronary blood flow by preventing arterial collapse.

## CARDIOVASCULAR PHARMACOLOGY

Medications that may be considered in the management of the stable patient with a narrow-QRS tachycardia include:

- Adenosine
- Verapamil
- Digoxin
- Beta-blockers
- Diltiazem

## CARDIOVASCULAR PHARMACOLOGY

The endotracheal dose of epinephrine is 2-2.5 times the IV dose (2-2.5 mg).

- To administer, draw up 2-2.5 mg of epinephrine 1:1000 solution and add normal saline for a total volume of 10 ml.

## CARDIOVASCULAR PHARMACOLOGY

- Pure beta-adrenergic stimulating agents do increase myocardial contractility and heart rate, however, another effect of beta-receptor stimulation is peripheral vasodilation.
- In cardiac arrest, vasodilation results in decreased coronary and cerebral perfusion which offsets any benefit that might be received from improved myocardial contractility and increased heart rate.

## CARDIOVASCULAR PHARMACOLOGY

Diltiazem (Cardizem) is a calcium channel blocker indicated in:

- multifocal atrial tachycardia
- atrial fibrillation and atrial flutter with a rapid ventricular response.

## CARDIOVASCULAR PHARMACOLOGY

Name three effects of norepinephrine administration.

## CARDIOVASCULAR PHARMACOLOGY

An 82 year old male has a blood pressure of 78/44. The patient suffered a massive anterior wall MI yesterday and is now in cardiogenic shock.

Dopamine is ordered for this patient. What is the rationale for this action?

## CARDIOVASCULAR PHARMACOLOGY

Name three situations in which the use of beta-blockers should be avoided.

## CARDIOVASCULAR PHARMACOLOGY

Name the first drug used in the management of:

- asystole
- ventricular fibrillation
- pulseless electrical activity
- pulseless ventricular tachycardia

## CARDIOVASCULAR PHARMACOLOGY

What is the recommended lidocaine dosing regimen for the stable patient in ventricular tachycardia with a pulse?

## CARDIOVASCULAR PHARMACOLOGY

A total of 2 mg/kg of lidocaine has been administered to a 57 year old patient with a wide-complex tachycardia of uncertain origin. The monitor now displays a sinus rhythm at 74 beats/minute.

Should you hang a lidocaine drip?

## CARDIOVASCULAR PHARMACOLOGY

Name the two most common side effects of bretylium administration when administered to the patient with a pulse.

## CARDIOVASCULAR PHARMACOLOGY

Describe the dosing schedule for administration of sublingual nitroglycerin.

## CARDIOVASCULAR PHARMACOLOGY

- Dopamine is the drug of choice for treatment of pump failure with a systolic blood pressure between 70 and 100 mm Hg.
- Dopamine administration should result in an increase in myocardial contractility and a subsequent increase in cardiac output.

## CARDIOVASCULAR PHARMACOLOGY

Norepinephrine possesses both alpha and beta-adrenergic receptor stimulating properties. Effects of administration may include:
- renal and mesenteric vasoconstriction
- peripheral vasoconstriction
- increase in heart rate
- increase in myocardial contractility.

## CARDIOVASCULAR PHARMACOLOGY

Epinephrine is the first drug administered to the patient with:
- asystole
- ventricular fibrillation
- pulseless electrical activity
- pulseless ventricular tachycardia.

## CARDIOVASCULAR PHARMACOLOGY

Beta-blockers should not be administered to patients with:
- hypotension
- bradycardia
- congestive heart failure
- second or third-degree AV block
- history of bronchospastic disease.

## CARDIOVASCULAR PHARMACOLOGY

- Yes. Prepare a continuous lidocaine infusion to run at 1 mg/minute more than the total bolus dose given.
- In this scenario, 2 mg/kg of lidocaine was administered by IV bolus. Begin administration of the lidocaine infusion at 3 mg/minute.

## CARDIOVASCULAR PHARMACOLOGY

- The initial lidocaine bolus is 1-1.5 mg/kg.
- The repeat dose is 1/2 the initial dose (0.5-0.75 mg/kg) every 5-10 minutes as needed to a maximum dose of 3 mg/kg.
- Prepare a lidocaine infusion.

## CARDIOVASCULAR PHARMACOLOGY

- One sublingual nitroglycerin tablet may be administered every 5 minutes to a maximum dose of 3 tablets.
- Monitor the patient's blood pressure closely before, during and after administration of the drug.

## CARDIOVASCULAR PHARMACOLOGY

The most common side effects of bretylium administration when administered to the patient with a pulse are:
- nausea and vomiting
- hypotension.

## CARDIOVASCULAR PHARMACOLOGY

Name three ACLS medications that stimulate beta-adrenergic receptors.

## CARDIOVASCULAR PHARMACOLOGY

Name two components of the ECG that should be monitored closely during the administration of procainamide.

## CARDIOVASCULAR PHARMACOLOGY

Name two situations in which sodium bicarbonate is considered a Class IIa (probably helpful) intervention.

## CARDIOVASCULAR PHARMACOLOGY

What are the most frequent complications of thrombolytic therapy?

## CARDIOVASCULAR PHARMACOLOGY

Name three calcium channel blockers.

## CARDIOVASCULAR PHARMACOLOGY

Explain why administration of endotracheal diazepam (Valium) is not recommended in the adult patient.

## CARDIOVASCULAR PHARMACOLOGY

Name four side effects of dopamine administration.

## CARDIOVASCULAR PHARMACOLOGY

Name three signs and symptoms of digitalis toxicity.

## CARDIOVASCULAR PHARMACOLOGY

When administering procainamide, monitor the ECG closely for:
- increasing PR intervals
- increasing QT intervals
  - may precipitate Torsades de Pointes
- widening of the QRS complex

## CARDIOVASCULAR PHARMACOLOGY

ACLS medications that stimulate beta-adrenergic receptors include:
- isoproterenol (pure beta-stimulator)
- dobutamine (pure beta-stimulator)
- norepinephrine (alpha & beta-stimulator)
- epinephrine (alpha & beta-stimulator)
- dopamine (dopaminergic, alpha & beta-stimulator)

## CARDIOVASCULAR PHARMACOLOGY

The most frequent complications of thrombolytic therapy are bleeding (particularly intracerebral hemorrhage) and dysrhythmias.
- Eisenberg MS, Aghababian RV, Bossaert L, Jaffe AS, Ornato JP, Weaver WD: Thrombolytic therapy, Ann Emerg Med 22:417-427, 1993.

## CARDIOVASCULAR PHARMACOLOGY

Sodium bicarbonate administration is considered a Class IIa (probably helpful) intervention:
- if overdose with cyclic antidepressants
- to alkalinize the urine in drug overdoses
- if known pre-existing bicarbonate-responsive acidosis

## CARDIOVASCULAR PHARMACOLOGY

- Diazepam is packaged as 10 mg in 2 ml. This volume is adequate for endotracheal administration in neonates and small children, however, is insufficient for endotracheal administration in the adult.
- The recommended minimum volume for adult endotracheal drug administration is 5 ml. Diazepam administration via this route would necessitate diluting it. Diazepam precipitates in normal saline and D5W and must be diluted with 95% ethanol. Diazepam administered via the endotracheal route has been associated with chemical pneumonitis and inflammation. Ethanol may cause deleterious changes in blood oxygenation.
  - Rusli M et al: Endotracheal diazepam: absorption and pulmonary pathologic effects, Ann Emerg Med. 16:314-318, 1987.

## CARDIOVASCULAR PHARMACOLOGY

The more common calcium channel blockers include:
- Verapamil (Isoptin, Calan)
- Nifedipine (Procardia, Adalat)
- Diltiazem (Cardizem)
- Nicardipine (Cardene)

## CARDIOVASCULAR PHARMACOLOGY

- The most common adverse effects of chronic digitalis toxicity are visual disturbances and fatigue. Visual disturbances include blurred vision, halos around solid objects and distorted perception of the colors red, yellow and green.
- Weakness
- Nausea, vomiting, loss of appetite, abdominal discomfort, diarrhea
- Dizziness, abnormal dreams, headache
- Cardiac toxicity:
  - SA block, sinus arrest, atrial fibrillation with a slow ventricular response, second or third-degree AV block, accelerated junctional rhythm, frequent uniform or multiformed PVCs, VT, atrial tachycardia with AV block.

## CARDIOVASCULAR PHARMACOLOGY

| | |
|---|---|
| CNS: | Headache, tremors |
| Cardiovascular: | Tachycardia, ventricular irritability (due to increased myocardial oxygen demand), palpitations |
| Other: | Nausea/vomiting; extravasation may cause tissue necrosis and sloughing<br>Vasodilation at low doses<br>Vasoconstriction at high doses |

## CARDIOVASCULAR PHARMACOLOGY

Describe the clinical effects of bretylium administration.

## CARDIOVASCULAR PHARMACOLOGY

Name two possible side effects of adenosine administration.

## CARDIOVASCULAR PHARMACOLOGY

Name two possible complications related to the administration of beta-blockers.

## CARDIOVASCULAR PHARMACOLOGY

Describe how to prepare a lidocaine infusion.

## CARDIOVASCULAR PHARMACOLOGY

How does lidocaine dosing differ for the patient in pulseless VT or VF from the patient in VT with a pulse, wide-complex tachycardia of uncertain origin or significant ventricular ectopy?

## CARDIOVASCULAR PHARMACOLOGY

Describe the mechanism of action of amrinone.

## CARDIOVASCULAR PHARMACOLOGY

In therapeutic doses, does lidocaine affect myocardial contractility?

## CARDIOVASCULAR PHARMACOLOGY

Stimulation of alpha receptor sites results in __.

## CARDIOVASCULAR PHARMACOLOGY

- Cardiovascular = facial flushing, headache, transient hypotension, chest pressure
  - development of transient torsades de pointes, followed by VT and cardiac arrest in a patient who received adenosine for PSVT has been reported
  - development of prolonged asystole (13-15 sec) following administration of adenosine for PSVT has been reported
  - development of marked acceleration of the ventricular response in rapid atrial fibrillation has been reported
- CNS = lightheadedness
- Respiratory = dyspnea
- GI = nausea

## CARDIOVASCULAR PHARMACOLOGY

- Bretylium initially causes a transient increase in heart rate, blood pressure, and peripheral vasoconstriction due to the release of norepinephrine.
- Approximately 15-20 minutes later, bretylium blocks the reuptake and further release of norepinephrine from sympathetic nerve endings (adrenergic blockade) which may result in significant hypotension.

## CARDIOVASCULAR PHARMACOLOGY

- To prepare a lidocaine infusion mix 1 gram of lidocaine in 250 ml of IV solution (or 2 grams in 500 ml).
- The infusion rate is usually 1 mg/minute more than the total bolus dose given. For example:
  - bolus 1 mg/kg — drip 2 mg/min
  - bolus 1 1/2-2 mg/kg — drip 3 mg/min
  - bolus 2 1/2-3 mg/kg — drip 4 mg/min
- The maintenance infusion rate is reduced to 1/2 the usual rate in patients > 70 years of age, in patients with signs of shock, hepatic dysfunction or in CHF.

## CARDIOVASCULAR PHARMACOLOGY

- Hypotension
- Bradydysrhythmias
- AV conduction delays
- Precipitation of bronchospasm
- Precipitation of congestive heart failure

## CARDIOVASCULAR PHARMACOLOGY

- Amrinone is a phosphodiesterase inhibitor. Phosphodiesterase is an enzyme that breaks down cyclic AMP (cAMP). Higher levels of cyclic AMP result due to inhibition of phosphodiesterase and the amount of calcium available for muscle contraction increases. The net result is an increased inotropic effect (myocardial contractility).
- Amrinone also relaxes vascular smooth muscle, resulting in vasodilation (decreasing afterload).

## CARDIOVASCULAR PHARMACOLOGY

- In pulseless VT or VF, the initial bolus of lidocaine is 1-1.5 mg/kg. You may rebolus with the same dose every 5 minutes to a maximum of 3 mg/kg.
- In VT with a pulse, wide-complex tachycardia of uncertain origin or in cases of significant ventricular ectopy, the initial bolus of lidocaine is 1-1.5 mg/kg but repeat doses of the drug are administered at 1/2 the initial dose every 5 minutes to a maximum of 3 mg/kg.

## CARDIOVASCULAR PHARMACOLOGY

Stimulation of alpha receptor sites results in peripheral vasoconstriction.

## CARDIOVASCULAR PHARMACOLOGY

In therapeutic doses, lidocaine does NOT significantly affect myocardial contractility.

## CARDIOVASCULAR PHARMACOLOGY

Name three sides effects of isoproterenol administration.

## CARDIOVASCULAR PHARMACOLOGY

Describe the mechanism of action of propranolol (Inderal).

## CARDIOVASCULAR PHARMACOLOGY

What is the recommended dose of aspirin for the patient experiencing an acute myocardial infarction?

## CARDIOVASCULAR PHARMACOLOGY

Explain why aspirin is recommended for administration at the earliest opportunity for the patient with new-onset chest pain whose origin is presumed to be due to ischemic heart disease.

## CARDIOVASCULAR PHARMACOLOGY

How is diltiazem administered for the patient with atrial fibrillation or atrial flutter with a rapid ventricular response?

## CARDIOVASCULAR PHARMACOLOGY

Name three medications that may be used for sedation and alleviation of pain prior to the delivery of electrical therapy in the conscious patient.

## CARDIOVASCULAR PHARMACOLOGY

Which of the following exert a positive inotropic effect?

- digitalis
- diltiazem
- dopamine

## CARDIOVASCULAR PHARMACOLOGY

- Propranolol is a nonselective beta-adrenergic blocker.
- Propranolol blocks beta-1 adrenergic receptors resulting in decreased heart rate, myocardial irritability, decreased force of contraction, and slowing of atrioventricular and intraventricular conduction velocity.
- By blocking catecholamine-induced increases in heart rate and blood pressure, propranolol decreases myocardial oxygen demand.

## CARDIOVASCULAR PHARMACOLOGY

- Cardiovascular:
  - Palpitations, tachycardia, possible extension of MI, cardiac dysrhythmias (including VT and VF), hypotension, angina
- CNS:
  - Nervousness, dizziness, anxiety, insomnia, weakness, mild tremor, headache
- Other:
  - Nausea/vomiting, sweating, flushing of the face or skin

## CARDIOVASCULAR PHARMACOLOGY

Administration of aspirin is thought to impede clotting by blocking prostaglandin synthesis in platelets. This prevents formation of thromboxane A2, a platelet-aggregating substance and prostaglandin derivative.

## CARDIOVASCULAR PHARMACOLOGY

- The recommended dose of aspirin is 150-325 mg (adult aspirin).
- Two to four 81 mg flavored children's aspirin are often substituted for the adult dose. The patient may be asked to chew the tablets to enhance absorption.

## CARDIOVASCULAR PHARMACOLOGY

- Sedatives:
  - Diazepam (Valium)
  - Midazolam (Versed)
  - Barbiturates
  - Etomidate (Amidate)
  - Ketamine (Ketalar)
  - Methohexital (Brevital sodium)
- Analgesics:
  - Fentanyl (Sublimaze)
  - Morphine
  - Meperidine (Demerol)

## CARDIOVASCULAR PHARMACOLOGY

- The initial dose is 0.25 mg/kg (20 mg) IV bolus over 2 minutes.
- If needed, a second IV bolus of 0.35 mg/kg (25 mg) may be administered over 2 minutes.
- Diltiazem may also be administered as a continuous IV infusion.
  - Mix 250 mg in 250 ml of IV solution.
  - The recommended initial infusion rate is 10 mg/hour.

## CARDIOVASCULAR PHARMACOLOGY

- Digitalis and dopamine strengthen or increase the force of myocardial contraction (positive inotropic effect).
- Diltiazem, a calcium channel blocker, exerts a negative inotropic effect (weakens or decreases the force of myocardial contraction).

## SPECIAL RESUSCITATION SITUATIONS

Name three factors that influence a drowning victim's chances for survival.

## SPECIAL RESUSCITATION SITUATIONS

Name three secondary injuries that may occur as a result of electrocution.

## SPECIAL RESUSCITATION SITUATIONS

A 65 year old male is suffering from hypothermia. He is unconscious and breathing very shallowly at a rate of 4-6 breaths per minute. His carotid pulse is barely palpable at 40 beats/minute.

How will you manage this patient's airway?

## SPECIAL RESUSCITATION SITUATIONS

Name three possible precipitants of cardiac arrest in the pregnant patient.

## SPECIAL RESUSCITATION SITUATIONS

Explain how aspiration of saltwater may result in pulmonary edema.

## SPECIAL RESUSCITATION SITUATIONS

Define "stroke."

## SPECIAL RESUSCITATION SITUATIONS

What is the most important forecaster of ischemic stroke?

## SPECIAL RESUSCITATION SITUATIONS

Describe Advanced Cardiac Life Support measures that should be instituted in the management of the victim of an electrocution.

## SPECIAL RESUSCITATION SITUATIONS

- Fractures
  - cervical spine
  - skull (due to fall, blunt trauma)
  - femur
  - humerus
- Closed head injury
- Myoglobinuria
- Peripheral nerve injury

## SPECIAL RESUSCITATION SITUATIONS

- Ability to swim
- Age of the victim
- Length of submersion
- Cleanliness of the water
- Temperature of the water
- Pre-existing medical conditions.

## SPECIAL RESUSCITATION SITUATIONS

- Trauma
- Myocardial infarction
- Pulmonary embolism
- Amniotic fluid embolism
- Congestive heart failure
- Congenital and acquired cardiac disease
- Peripartum hemorrhage with hypovolemia

## SPECIAL RESUSCITATION SITUATIONS

- This patient is not ventilating adequately.
- Ventilate the patient with 100% oxygen with a bag-valve-mask and prepare to intubate.
  - "Endotracheal intubation to provide effective ventilation with warm, humidified oxygen and to prevent aspiration should be performed in the unconscious hypothermic patient with inadequate ventilation."
    - Emergency Cardiac Care Committee and Subcommittees, American Heart Association. Guidelines for cardiopulmonary resuscitation and emergency cardiac care, JAMA 268:2245, 1992.

## SPECIAL RESUSCITATION SITUATIONS

An illness of sudden onset caused by occlusion or rupture of a blood vessel in the brain.

## SPECIAL RESUSCITATION SITUATIONS

Saltwater is hypertonic and results in shifting of intravascular fluid into the alveoli.

## SPECIAL RESUSCITATION SITUATIONS

- VF, asystole and other serious dysrhythmias should be treated per the ACLS guidelines for these rhythms.
- Intubate
  - Intubation may be difficult with electrical burns of the face, mouth or anterior neck due to soft-tissue swelling.
- Rapid IV fluid administration if hypovolemic shock or significant tissue destruction is present.
  - Counteracts shock
  - Corrects ongoing fluids losses
  - Maintains a diuresis to avoid renal shutdown due to myoglobinuria

## SPECIAL RESUSCITATION SITUATIONS

The most important forecaster of ischemic stroke is the occurrence of a transient ischemic attack (TIA).

## SPECIAL RESUSCITATION SITUATIONS

Should the Heimlich maneuver be routinely used as a first-step in the management of all victims of near-drowning?

## SPECIAL RESUSCITATION SITUATIONS

Define the term "transient ischemic attack."

## SPECIAL RESUSCITATION SITUATIONS

Define "immersion syndrome."

## SPECIAL RESUSCITATION SITUATIONS

What is meant by the term "after-drop" phenomenon?

## SPECIAL RESUSCITATION SITUATIONS

Name three signs and symptoms of moderate hypothermia.

## SPECIAL RESUSCITATION SITUATIONS

What is supine hypotension?

## SPECIAL RESUSCITATION SITUATIONS

Name two injuries that may be associated with a near-drowning incident.

## SPECIAL RESUSCITATION SITUATIONS

Name three signs of a stroke.

## SPECIAL RESUSCITATION SITUATIONS

A transient ischemic attack (TIA) is a reversible episode of focal neurologic dysfunction (such as a speech disorder, weakness, paralysis) lasting a few minutes to hours but resolving within 24 hours.

## SPECIAL RESUSCITATION SITUATIONS

No. The Heimlich maneuver should be reserved for situations in which airway obstruction due to the presence of a foreign body is suspected or when the victim does not respond to mouth-to-mouth ventilation.

## SPECIAL RESUSCITATION SITUATIONS

- After-drop phenomenon may occur as a result of external rewarming of the hypothermic patient, which leads to peripheral vasodilation. "After-drop" refers to a drop in core temperature as cold blood is returned from the peripheral circulation to the central circulation.
- After-drop phenomenon may be fatal.

## SPECIAL RESUSCITATION SITUATIONS

Delayed sudden death triggered by vagally induced dysrhythmias after cold water immersion.

## SPECIAL RESUSCITATION SITUATIONS

- Supine hypotension is a common complication of late pregnancy which results when the gravid uterus compresses the abdominal aorta and inferior vena cava, reducing venous return to the heart.
- Supine hypotension is defined as a mean blood pressure decrease of 15 mm Hg and a sustained increase in the pulse rate of 20 beats per minute.
- Positioning the pregnant female on her left side may increase cardiac output by 25% (Brinkman and Woods, 1979).

## SPECIAL RESUSCITATION SITUATIONS

- No shivering
- Decreased reflexes
- Bradydysrhythmias, PVCs
- Decreased respiratory rate
- Increased muscular rigidity
- Progressive decrease in level of consciousness

## SPECIAL RESUSCITATION SITUATIONS

Signs of a stroke may include:

- Coma
- Ataxia
- Incoordination
- Facial asymmetry
- Inability to speak
- Incoherent speech
- Visual disturbances
- Altered level of consciousness

## SPECIAL RESUSCITATION SITUATIONS

- Hypothermia
- Spinal cord injury (diving)
- Air embolism or the "bends" (SCUBA)

## SPECIAL RESUSCITATION SITUATIONS

Name two signs and symptoms of severe hypothermia.

## SPECIAL RESUSCITATION SITUATIONS

What is the preferred IV solution for administration in the emergency treatment of suspected stroke?

## SPECIAL RESUSCITATION SITUATIONS

Name four possible causes of traumatic cardiac arrest.

## SPECIAL RESUSCITATION SITUATIONS

A 35 year old pregnant (30 weeks) female has suffered a cardiac arrest. The cardiac monitor displays ventricular fibrillation.

How will you manage this resuscitation effort?

## SPECIAL RESUSCITATION SITUATIONS

Define "ischemic stroke."

## SPECIAL RESUSCITATION SITUATIONS

Name three basic life support interventions that should be initiated in the severely hypothermic patient.

## SPECIAL RESUSCITATION SITUATIONS

Why is alternating current more damaging than direct current?

## SPECIAL RESUSCITATION SITUATIONS

Name two possible underlying causes of a near-drowning incident.

## SPECIAL RESUSCITATION SITUATIONS

- The preferred IV solution in suspected stroke is normal saline or lactated Ringer's solution.
- Avoid D5W unless hypoglycemia is STRONGLY suspected.
  - D5W is hypotonic and may increase cerebral edema.

## SPECIAL RESUSCITATION SITUATIONS

- Rigidity
- Hypotension
- Stupor, coma
- Eventual VF or asystole
- Undetectable pulse and respiration

## SPECIAL RESUSCITATION SITUATIONS

- CPR until a defibrillator is available
- Defibrillate as needed with 200, 200-300, 360J
- Intubate
- IV access
- Displace the uterus to the left
- Pharmacologic therapy WITHOUT any modifications
- Prompt cesarean section should be considered if the above measures have failed to restore effective circulation.

## SPECIAL RESUSCITATION SITUATIONS

- Severe central neurological injury with secondary cardiovascular collapse
- Direct and severe injury to vital structures (heart, aorta)
- Severely diminished oxygen delivery
- Injuries in a cold environment complicated (e.g., fractured leg) by secondary severe hypothermia
- Underlying medical problems that led to the injury (such as sudden VF)
- Hypoxia secondary to respiratory arrest resulting from neurological injury, airway obstruction, large open pneumothorax or severe tracheobronchial laceration or crush.

## SPECIAL RESUSCITATION SITUATIONS

- If apneic, initiate rescue breathing
- If pulseless, initiate CPR
  - Pulse and respirations may need to be checked for 30-45 seconds to confirm pulselessness or profound bradycardia
- Administer warm, humidified oxygen
- Remove wet garments
- Protect against heat loss and wind chill
- Maintain horizontal position
- Avoid rough movement and excess activity.

## SPECIAL RESUSCITATION SITUATIONS

An artery is blocked by a blood clot that either developed within the vessel (thrombosis) or arose from another source (such as the heart) and travelled to the brain (embolism).

- Accounts for approximately 75% of strokes

## SPECIAL RESUSCITATION SITUATIONS

- Seizures
- Hypoglycemia
- Suicide, homicide or child abuse
- Alcohol or other substance ingestion

## SPECIAL RESUSCITATION SITUATIONS

Alternating current (household and industrial current) is three times more damaging than direct current because of its ability to:

- cause tetanic muscle contractions
- "freeze" the victim to the circuit.

## SPECIAL RESUSCITATION SITUATIONS

Define "hemorrhagic stroke."

## SPECIAL RESUSCITATION SITUATIONS

Name three interventions that may be instituted in the management of increased intracranial pressure associated with suspected stroke.

## SPECIAL RESUSCITATION SITUATIONS

Of the following pathways of electrical current, which is most likely to be fatal?

- foot-to-foot
- hand-to-foot
- hand-to-hand

## SPECIAL RESUSCITATION SITUATIONS

Describe the interventions that should be instituted in the pre-hospital management of cardiac arrest due to hypothermia.

## SPECIAL RESUSCITATION SITUATIONS

Name three symptoms of a stroke.

## SPECIAL RESUSCITATION SITUATIONS

What is the rationale for hyper-ventilating the patient with increased intracranial pressure?

## SPECIAL RESUSCITATION SITUATIONS

Describe basic life support management of the moderately hypothermic patient.

## SPECIAL RESUSCITATION SITUATIONS

Name three signs and symptoms of mild hypothermia.

## SPECIAL RESUSCITATION SITUATIONS

- Fluid restriction
- Elevate the head of the bed
- Intubate and hyperventilate to a PCO2 of 25-28 mm Hg
- Control of agitation and pain
- Mannitol 1-2 g/kg IV over 5-10 min

## SPECIAL RESUSCITATION SITUATIONS

- Hemorrhagic stroke is the result of a ruptured cerebral blood vessel.
- Bleeding can occur adjacent to the brain (subarachnoid hemorrhage) or bleeding can occur into the substance of the brain (intracerebral hemorrhage).

## SPECIAL RESUSCITATION SITUATIONS

- Initiate CPR
- If VF or pulseless VT, defibrillate with 200, 300, 360J as needed
- Intubate
- Ventilate with warm, humidified oxygen
- Establish IV
- Infuse warm normal saline
- If the patient fails to respond to initial defibrillation attempts, (limit to three) or drug therapy, withhold further shocks and transport to the hospital.

## SPECIAL RESUSCITATION SITUATIONS

The hand-to-hand (transthoracic) pathway is more likely to be fatal than the hand-to-foot (vertical) or foot-to-foot (straddle) pathway.

- The hand-to-foot pathway may cause myocardial injury but is associated with a lower mortality and fewer complications.

## SPECIAL RESUSCITATION SITUATIONS

Hyperventilation is an effective, although temporary, measure that helps to reduce increased intracranial pressure by blowing off excess carbon dioxide.

## SPECIAL RESUSCITATION SITUATIONS

- Weakness
- Confusion
- Photophobia
- Hearing loss
- Double vision
- Intense vertigo
- Nausea/vomiting
- Facial weakness
- Intense or unusually severe headache

## SPECIAL RESUSCITATION SITUATIONS

- Shivering
- Memory loss
- Poor judgment
- Pale, cold, dry skin
- Lack of coordination
- Early rise in blood pressure and respiratory rates

## SPECIAL RESUSCITATION SITUATIONS

- Administer warm, humidified oxygen.
- Apply warm packs to the neck, axilla and groin.
- Transport cautiously and gently.

## SPECIAL RESUSCITATION SITUATIONS

The Glasgow Coma Scale is a tool that may be used to assess the severity of neurologic deficit in the patient experiencing a suspected stroke.

What areas are evaluated when using the Glasgow Coma Scale?

## SPECIAL RESUSCITATION SITUATIONS

When discussing the effects of current intensity with electrical injuries, 5-30 milliamps is described as the "let go current."

What is meant by this phrase?

## SPECIAL RESUSCITATION SITUATIONS

Explain how respiratory arrest may occur as a result of an electrical injury.

## SPECIAL RESUSCITATION SITUATIONS

If stroke is suspected, at what rate should intravenous solutions be infused?

## SPECIAL RESUSCITATION SITUATIONS

Name five signs and symptoms of cocaine overdose.

## SPECIAL RESUSCITATION SITUATIONS

Name four situations not initially involving the heart that may cause cardiac arrest.

## SPECIAL RESUSCITATION SITUATIONS

Name four factors that determine the impact of electrical injuries.

## SPECIAL RESUSCITATION SITUATIONS

What is the primary concern in the management of the near-drowning victim?

## SPECIAL RESUSCITATION SITUATIONS

- Within a current range of 5-30 milliamps, the victim is usually able to "let go" of the current source.
- Beyond this range, the presence of involuntary muscle contractions make it impossible for the victim to "let go" of the current source.

## SPECIAL RESUSCITATION SITUATIONS

The Glasgow Coma Scale is used to assess:
- eye opening
- motor response
- verbal response

## SPECIAL RESUSCITATION SITUATIONS

- An IV solution of normal saline or lactated Ringer's should be infused at a rate of 30 ml/hour.
- Unless the patient is hypotensive, rapid infusions should be avoided due to the risk of increased intracranial pressure.

## SPECIAL RESUSCITATION SITUATIONS

Respiratory arrest may occur secondary to:
- electric current passing through the brain and causing inhibition of medullary respiratory center function
- tetanic contraction of the diaphragm and chest wall musculature during current exposure
- prolonged paralysis of the respiratory muscles may continue for minutes after the electric shock has terminated.

## SPECIAL RESUSCITATION SITUATIONS

- Stroke
- Trauma
- Pregnancy
- Hypothermia
- Near-drowning
- Electrical shock/lightning strike

## SPECIAL RESUSCITATION SITUATIONS

- Dyspnea
- Seizures
- Tachycardia
- Hypertension
- Hyperthermia
- Agitation, confusion
- Chest pain, acute MI
- Respiratory depression/arrest

## SPECIAL RESUSCITATION SITUATIONS

- Major physiological consequences of near-drowning include acidosis, hypoxemia and the development of pulmonary edema.
- Of these, hypoxemia is the most important.

## SPECIAL RESUSCITATION SITUATIONS

- Voltage
- Amperage
- Type of current
- Pathway of current
- Resistance of tissues
- Duration of exposure to current

## PUTTING IT ALL TOGETHER

A 52 year old male states he feels his "heart is racing." When questioned, he denies chest pain or difficulty breathing. The cardiac monitor displays ventricular tachycardia at 180 beats/minute. His blood pressure is 130/74, respiratory rate 16.

How will you manage this patient?

## PUTTING IT ALL TOGETHER

A 36 year old female is complaining of palpitations. She is awake and denies chest pain or difficulty breathing. Examination reveals a blood pressure of 144/82 and a respiratory rate of 14-16 breaths/minute. The cardiac monitor displays a narrow-QRS tachycardia at a rate of 180 beats/minute.

Name three medications that should be considered in the management of this patient.

## PUTTING IT ALL TOGETHER

Name five possible causes of pulseless electrical activity.

## PUTTING IT ALL TOGETHER

A 62 year old male is complaining of severe mid-chest pain radiating to his left arm and jaw. His blood pressure is 74/48, respiratory rate 18. The cardiac monitor displays a sinus bradycardia at 38 beats/minute with frequent, multiformed PVCs.

Describe your management of this patient.

## PUTTING IT ALL TOGETHER

A 74 year old male is complaining of chest pain, nausea and general weakness. The cardiac monitor displays a second-degree AV block, type I at 44-50 beats/minute. The patient's blood pressure is 62/40, respiratory rate 16. Breath sounds are clear. The patient is awake but pale, diaphoretic and anxious.

How will you manage this patient?

## PUTTING IT ALL TOGETHER

Name the first antidysrhythmic administered in the management of the patient in ventricular fibrillation.

## PUTTING IT ALL TOGETHER

Name three medications that may be considered in the management of the patient in atrial fibrillation or atrial flutter with a rapid ventricular response.

## PUTTING IT ALL TOGETHER

- You are a paramedic called to a private residence for an "ill woman." You arrive to find a 46 year old female lying face down on her bed. The patient's sister states that 15 minutes before she called you, the patient said she couldn't breathe and needed someone to take her to the hospital. The patient has a history of CHF and asthma and takes 30 mg of Procardia and 0.25 mg of Lanoxin daily.
- You find the patient to be pulseless and apneic. The cardiac monitor displays the rhythm below. Examination of the patient reveals no sign of trauma.
- How will you manage this patient?

Lead II

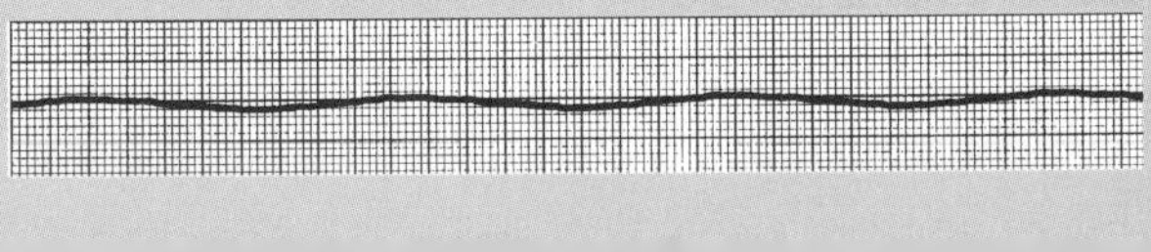

## PUTTING IT ALL TOGETHER

The patient described in clinically stable. Management of the stable patient with a narrow-QRS tachycardia should include consideration of the following medications:

- Adenosine
- Verapamil
- Digoxin
- Beta-blockers
- Diltiazem

## PUTTING IT ALL TOGETHER

- This patient is clinically stable. Administer oxygen, establish an IV and administer lidocaine 1-1.5 mg/kg IV bolus.
- Repeat with 0.5-0.75 mg/kg as needed every 5 minutes to a maximum dose of 3 mg/kg.
- If the dysrhythmia is resolved with lidocaine, prepare a lidocaine infusion.

## PUTTING IT ALL TOGETHER

- Administer oxygen and establish IV access.
- Administer atropine 0.5-1.0 mg RAPID IV bolus and reassess.
- Administration of medications for pain relief should be withheld until the patient's systolic blood pressure is 100 mm Hg.
- If the patient's heart rate increases above 60 beats/minute and significant ventricular ectopy exists, consider lidocaine administration.
- Administer aspirin (if not contraindicated) and evaluate the patient for possible thrombolytic therapy.

## PUTTING IT ALL TOGETHER

Possible causes of pulseless electrical activity may be remembered by the use of MATCH(x4)ED:

- Myocardial infarction (massive)
- Acidosis
- Tension pneumothorax
- Cardiac tamponade
- Hypovolemia (most common cause)
- Hypoxia
- Hypothermia
- Hyperkalemia
- Embolism (massive pulmonary)
- Drug overdose (cyclic antidepressants, digitalis, beta-blockers, calcium channel blockers)

## PUTTING IT ALL TOGETHER

The first antidysrhythmic administered in the treatment of VF is lidocaine.

## PUTTING IT ALL TOGETHER

- Administer oxygen and establish IV access.
- Administer atropine 0.5-1.0 mg RAPID IV bolus and reassess. This dose may be repeated every 3-5 minutes as needed to a maximum dose of 2-3 mg.
- Transcutaneous pacing may be considered if atropine administration proves unsuccessful.
- A 200-250 ml fluid challenge may be administered to rule out hypovolemia. If no response, consider dopamine administration (5-20 mcg/kg/min).
- An epinephrine infusion (2-10 mcg/min) may be considered.
- Isoproterenol (LOW dose) may be considered if other measures have proven unsuccessful.

## PUTTING IT ALL TOGETHER

- Initiate CPR -
- Confirm the rhythm in another lead
- Intubate (confirm tube placement)
- Establish IV access with normal saline or lactated Ringer's solution
- Consider possible causes of this situation (Hx4AD)
    - Hypoxia, Hypokalemia, Hypothermia, Hyperkalemia, Acidosis (preexisting), Drug overdose
- Consider immediate transcutaneous pacing
- Administer epinephrine 1 mg IV bolus
    - May repeat every 3-5 minutes
- Administer atropine 1 mg IV bolus
    - May repeat with same dose every 3-5 min to a maximum of 3 mg

## PUTTING IT ALL TOGETHER

Management of the stable patient with atrial fibrillation or atrial flutter with a RAPID ventricular response may include:

- For rate control:
    - Beta-blockers (Esmolol, Propranolol, Metoprolol)
    - Calcium channel blockers (Diltiazem, Verapamil)
    - Digoxin
- For pharmacologic conversion:
    - Procainamide
    - Quinidine

## PUTTING IT ALL TOGETHER

The patient exhibiting signs and symptoms of acute pulmonary edema should be placed in a sitting position with the legs dependent.

Why might positioning of the patient in this manner prove beneficial?

## PUTTING IT ALL TOGETHER

Name, in order, the medication regimen (including dosages) for the stable patient with a wide-complex tachycardia of uncertain origin.

## PUTTING IT ALL TOGETHER

This 57 year old male is complaining of severe chest pain. On a scale of 1-10, he ranks his pain an 8. His blood pressure is 74/50. Breath sounds are clear. Respiratory rate is 14/minute.
How will you manage him?
Lead II

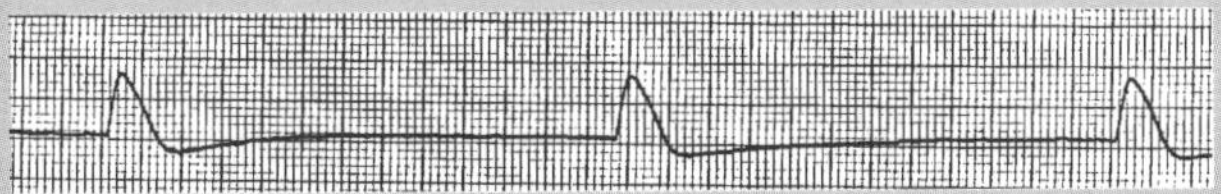

## PUTTING IT ALL TOGETHER

Name the medications that may be used in the management of the symptomatic patient with a narrow-QRS bradycardia.

## PUTTING IT ALL TOGETHER

This 45 year old female is complaining her "heart is racing." She denies chest pain or difficulty breathing although she is anxious and feels "lightheaded." Her blood pressure is 148/88, respiratory rate 18. Breath sounds are clear.
How will you manage her?
Lead II

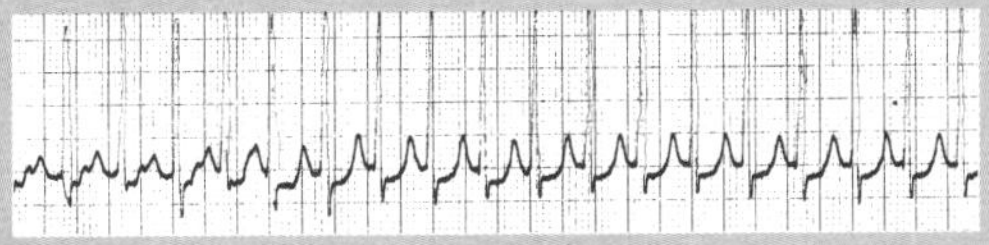

## PUTTING IT ALL TOGETHER

You have been called to a patient's room in which a code arrest is in progress. You find a 43 year old male unconscious, pulseless and apneic. CPR is being properly performed by a nurse and respiratory therapist. As the code cart is wheeled into the room, you perform a quick-look and see the rhythm below on the monitor.
Describe your initial management of this patient.
Lead II

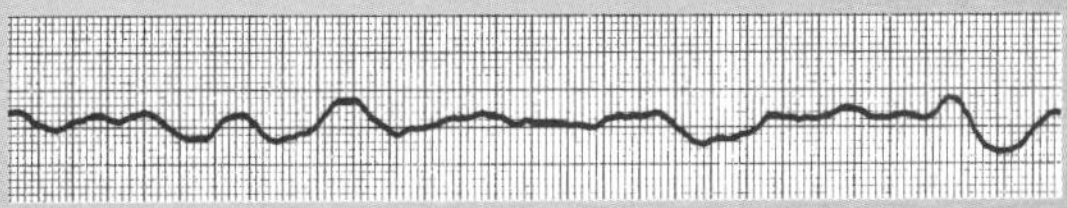

## PUTTING IT ALL TOGETHER

When is ventricular fibrillation or pulseless ventricular tachycardia termed "refractory" or "persistent"?

## PUTTING IT ALL TOGETHER

A 62 year old male is complaining of severe chest pain radiating to his left arm and a feeling of weakness. He is pale and diaphoretic. His history is significant for an anterior wall MI six weeks ago. Breath sounds are clear. BP 72/40, respirations 12.
How will you manage this patient?

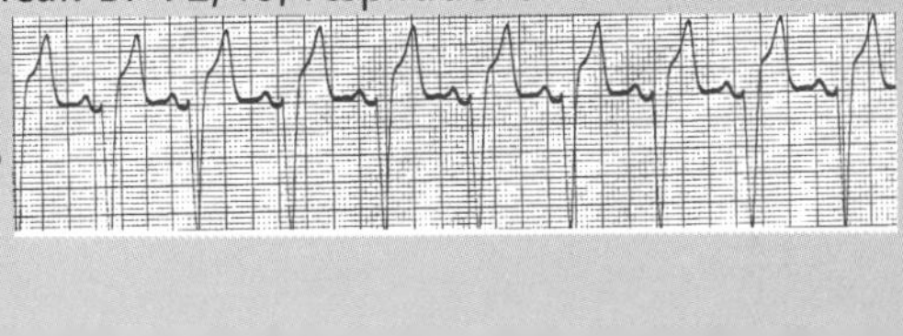

## PUTTING IT ALL TOGETHER

- Lidocaine
  - 1-1.5 mg/kg; may repeat with half this dose every 5 minutes to a maximum of 3 mg/kg
- Adenosine
  - 6 mg initial bolus; may repeat with 12 mg in 1-2 minutes if no response; may repeat 12 mg dose once in 1-2 minutes (total dose 30 mg)
- Procainamide
  - 20-30 mg/minute to a maximum dose of 17 mg/kg
- Bretylium
  - 5-10 mg/kg (dose injected into a 50 ml bag of solution and infused over 8-10 min)
  - Maximum dose 30 mg/kg over 24 hours.

## PUTTING IT ALL TOGETHER

Placing the patient experiencing acute pulmonary edema in a sitting position with the legs dependent:

- decreases the work of respiration
- decreases venous return to the heart
- increases lung volume and vital capacity

## PUTTING IT ALL TOGETHER

Medications that may be considered in the management of symptomatic narrow-QRS bradycardia are:

- Atropine (bolus)
- Dopamine (infusion)
- Epinephrine (infusion)
- Isoproterenol (infusion - LOW dose)

## PUTTING IT ALL TOGETHER

- The rhythm shown is an idioventricular (ventricular escape) rhythm.
- Administer oxygen, establish IV access and prepare for transcutaneous pacing.
- Medications for pain relief should be withheld until the patient's systolic blood pressure is at least 100 mm Hg.

## PUTTING IT ALL TOGETHER

- Visually confirming the rhythm on the cardiac monitor between shocks, defibrillate with 200, 200-300, 360J.
- Resume CPR
- Ask that the patient be intubated.
  - Hyperventilate prior to attempting the procedure, assure the attempt does not exceed 30 seconds and confirm tube placement upon completion of the procedure.
- Establish IV access (normal saline or lactated Ringer's solution).
- Administer epinephrine by the first medication route available.
  - 1 mg (1:10,000 solution) if IV available first
  - 2-2.5 mg (of 1:1000 solution diluted to a total volume of 10 ml of normal saline) if endotracheal tube placed first
- Defibrillate within 30-60 seconds.
- Reassess - is there a pulse?

## PUTTING IT ALL TOGETHER

- The rhythm is a supraventricular tachycardia (narrow-QRS tachycardia). This patient is clinically stable.
- Administer oxygen, establish IV access and perform a vagal maneuver (ask the patient to cough, bear down, etc.).
- If these maneuvers are unsuccessful, administer adenosine 6 mg rapid IV bolus.
- If the patient's rhythm and condition remain unchanged, administer adenosine 12 mg rapid IV bolus 1-2 minutes after the initial dose. The 12 mg bolus may be repeated once in 1-2 minutes if needed.

## PUTTING IT ALL TOGETHER

- The rhythm shown is a sinus rhythm with elevated ST segments.
- This patient is hypotensive. The key question is: Are the patient's signs and symptoms due to a rate problem, pump problem or volume problem? The patient's history and present signs and symptoms strongly suggest cardiogenic shock (pump problem).
- Administer oxygen and establish IV access. A 200-250 ml fluid challenge may be considered to rule out hypovolemia while preparations are made to administer a dopamine infusion.
  - Dopamine is the drug of choice for hypotension with a systolic blood pressure between 70 and 100 mm Hg.

## PUTTING IT ALL TOGETHER

VF or pulseless VT that persists after CPR, intubation, ventilation, four defibrillations and one or more doses of epinephrine is considered "refractory" or "persistent."

## PUTTING IT ALL TOGETHER

This patient is complaining of severe, crushing, mid-chest pain which has been present for 45 minutes with no relief from nitroglycerin. He has a past medical history of an MI 4 years ago, hypertension and angina. His blood pressure is 110/70, respirations 18.
How will you manage him?
Lead II

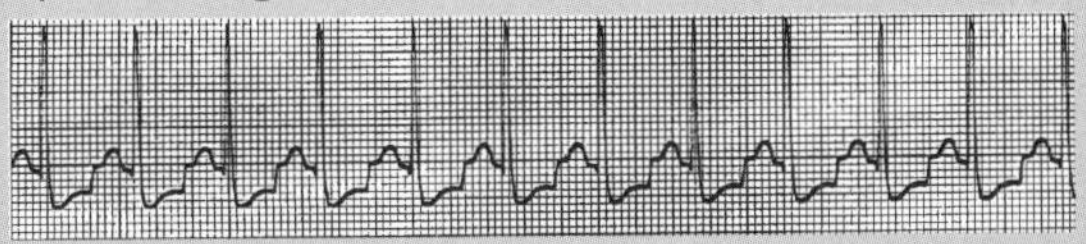

## PUTTING IT ALL TOGETHER

This 60 year old male is complaining of severe mid-chest pain present for 1 hour and dizziness. His blood pressure is 60/40, pulse rate is approximately 40 and respirations 14 per minute.
How will you manage this patient?
Lead II

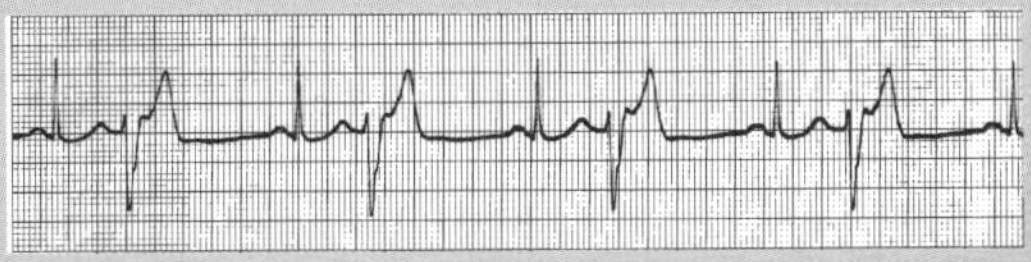

## PUTTING IT ALL TOGETHER

This 62 year old male has arrived in the Emergency Department complaining of palpitations. He states he was watching television when he felt a "fluttering" in his chest. He denies chest pain and difficulty breathing. He is awake and alert, but anxious. His blood pressure is 150/84, respirations 16. He has no significant past medical history and takes no medications regularly.
How will you manage this patient?
Lead II

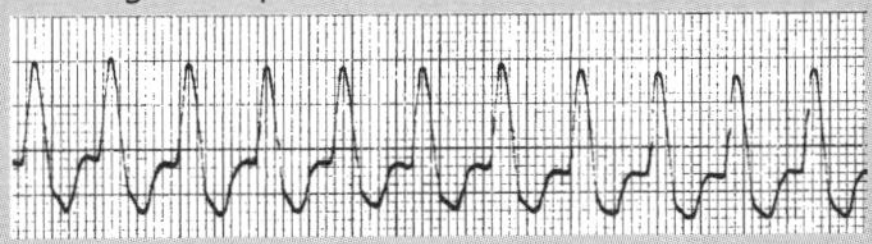

## PUTTING IT ALL TOGETHER

This is a 55 year old female complaining of chest pain radiating down her left arm. She is awake and alert with a blood pressure of 144/80 and a respiratory rate of 14-16/minute.
How will you manage this patient?
Lead II

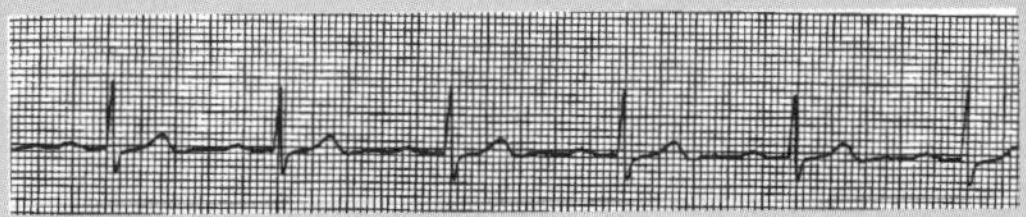

## PUTTING IT ALL TOGETHER

- It is 4:30 p.m. when a 66 year old female arrives in the Emergency Department. The patient is conscious and alert complaining of a sudden onset of weakness and numbness on her right side. The patient states she has had a "bad pain" in her head all day. The patient has a history of hypertension, a CVA 3 years ago, bypass surgery 5 years ago and seizures. The patient's medications include Quinidine, Methyldopa, Phenobarbital, Visken, Nitroglycerin and Meclizine.
- Examination reveals breath sounds are clear and equal bilaterally with a respiratory rate of 28. The abdomen is soft and nontender. There is equal movement and sensation in all extremities. The skin is warm and dry. Pupils are equal and reactive to light. Vital signs reveal a blood pressure of 240/120 and a pulse of 72 beats per minute, strong and regular. The cardiac monitor displays a sinus rhythm without ectopy.
- How will you manage this patient?

## PUTTING IT ALL TOGETHER

- A 58 year old female is complaining of dizziness and difficulty breathing. Her blood pressure is 64/40, respiratory rate 38-40 and labored. Breath sounds reveal bilateral crackles. Peripheral edema of the lower extremities is present to the patient's mid-calf. The patient's skin is cool and clammy. She has a history of CHF and normally takes Lanoxin and Lasix daily, however, due to a lack of transportation she has been unable to have her prescriptions refilled since she ran out of meds 12 days ago.
- How will you manage this patient?

Lead II

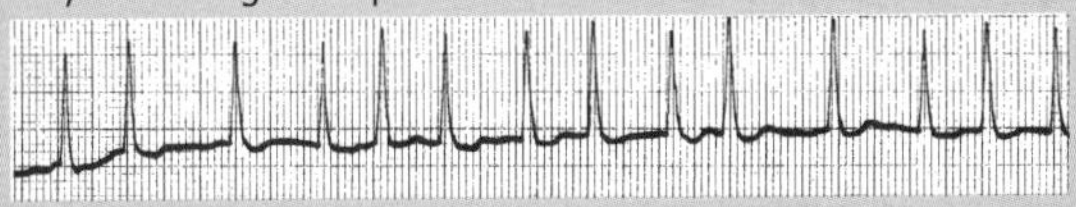

## PUTTING IT ALL TOGETHER

- An 82 year old female is complaining of difficulty breathing. The patient states she has had problems breathing all day but it has gotten progressively worse so her husband brought her to the Emergency Department. The patient is speaking in 4-5 word sentences.
- The pupils are equal and reactive to light. Auscultation of the chest reveals crackles bilaterally in the bases, clear breath sounds in the upper lobes. The abdomen is soft and nontender, no masses noted. The pelvis is intact. Movement and sensation is present in all extremities. Edema of the lower extremities is noted to the level of the mid-calf.
- The cardiac monitor displays a sinus tachycardia at 120 beats/minute. Initial vital signs reveals a blood pressure of 160/78, pulse of 120 (strong and regular) and a respiratory rate of 38 breaths per minute. The skin is cool and dry.
- The patient has a past medical history of CHF and a "mild heart condition." Medications include potassium, Lanoxin 0.25 mg daily, Prednisone and Lasix 40 mg daily.
- Describe your management of this patient.

## PUTTING IT ALL TOGETHER

- A 54 year old female is complaining of abdominal pain. She states the pain has been present for the past 3 hours and describes it as a "cramping" pain.
- Examination reveals the patient to be awake and alert. Pupils are equal and reactive to light. Lungs are clear bilaterally with a respiratory rate of 28 per minute. The right lower quadrant of the abdomen is tender to palpation. The abdomen is not distended and no masses are palpated. Motor function and sensation is normal in all extremities.
- The initial blood pressure is 72/P, pulse 120 (weak but regular) and respirations 28. The cardiac monitor shows a sinus tachycardia without ectopy.
- The patient has a history of lymphoma and had a splenectomy 1 year ago. Medications include Prednisone and Tagamet.
- How will you manage this patient?

## PUTTING IT ALL TOGETHER

- Administer oxygen.
- Establish IV access with normal saline and infuse at 30 ml/hour.
- Continuous ECG monitoring, obtain 12-lead ECG, pulse oximetry
- Portable chest roentgenogram
- Laboratory studies including: electrolytes, glucose, CBC and coagulation studies, ABGs
- Assess Glasgow Coma Scale
- Neuro consult
- CT of the brain without contrast.
  - Results of CT may help guide decision regarding the management of the patient's elevated blood pressure

## PUTTING IT ALL TOGETHER

- The rhythm shown is a sinus tachycardia with depressed ST segments and inverted T waves.
- Administer oxygen, establish IV access.
- Administer medication for pain relief.
- Administer aspirin (if not contraindicated).
- Determine if the patient is a candidate for thrombolytic therapy.

## PUTTING IT ALL TOGETHER

- The rhythm shown is atrial fibrillation with a rapid ventricular response.
- The patient is unstable as evidenced by significant hypotension and signs of congestive heart failure.
- Administer oxygen and establish IV access.
- Administer sedation and perform synchronized countershock with 100, 200, 300 and 360J as needed.
- Check pulses and reevaluate the patient's rhythm and condition between each shock!

## PUTTING IT ALL TOGETHER

- The rhythm shown is a sinus bradycardia with ventricular bigeminy.
- Administer oxygen and establish IV access.
- This patient is hypotensive. The key question to be asked is: Are the patient's signs and symptoms due to a rate problem, pump problem or volume problem?
- Assuming the patient's presentation is due to his significant bradycardia, administer atropine 0.5-1.0 mg RAPID IV bolus and reassess.
- Administration of medications for pain relief should be withheld until the patient's systolic blood pressure is 100 mm Hg.
- If the patient's heart rate increases above 60 beats/minute and significant ventricular ectopy exists, consider lidocaine administration.
- Administer aspirin (if not contraindicated) and evaluate the patient for possible thrombolytic therapy.

## PUTTING IT ALL TOGETHER

- Sit the patient up with legs dependent
- Administer oxygen, establish IV access and infuse at a to keep open (TKO) rate
- Continuous ECG monitoring, obtain 12-lead ECG, pulse oximetry, portable chest roentgenogram
- Administer sublingual nitroglycerin and reassess
- Administer furosemide 0.5-1.0 mg/kg IV bolus over 2 minutes
  - The patient regularly takes 40 mg of Lasix daily. This patient's physician opted to administer an initial dose of 80 mg.
- Consider morphine administration (1-3 mg) every 5 minutes titrated to effect.

## PUTTING IT ALL TOGETHER

- The rhythm shown is a wide-complex tachycardia and the patient appears clinically stable.
- Administer oxygen and establish IV access.
- The rhythm should first be treated as if it is ventricular tachycardia, therefore, the first drug that will be administered is lidocaine.
- Initial bolus 1-1.5 mg/kg. If needed, repeat with 1/2 the initial dose (0.5-0.75 mg/kg) every 5 minutes to a maximum of 3 mg/kg.
- If lidocaine therapy is unsuccessful, the rhythm should be treated as if it is supraventricular in origin. The drug that will be administered is adenosine.
- Initial bolus is 6 mg RAPID IV bolus. If needed, repeat with 12 mg in 1-2 minutes. The 12 mg dose may be repeated once in 1-2 minutes if needed.

## PUTTING IT ALL TOGETHER

- Administer oxygen and establish IV access.
- This patient is hypotensive and the cardiac monitor shows a sinus tachycardia at 120 beats/minute. The key question that should be asked is: Are the patient's signs and symptoms due to a rate problem, a pump problem, or a volume problem?
- The patient's breath sounds are clear. Administer a 200-250 ml fluid challenge and reevaluate the patient's condition.

## PUTTING IT ALL TOGETHER

- The rhythm shown is a sinus rhythm with a first-degree AV block.
- Administer oxygen and establish IV access.
- Administer medications for relief of pain.
- Administer aspirin (if not contraindicated) and evaluate the patient for possible thrombolytic therapy.
- Monitor the ECG closely for signs of increasing AV block.

## PUTTING IT ALL TOGETHER

- Paramedics are on the scene of a 56 year old male found unresponsive, pulseless and apneic. Police officers, first on the scene, are performing adequate CPR. The patient's past medical history is unobtainable, however the patient is wearing a nitropatch on the left upper chest and Nitrostat tablets were found on the kitchen counter.
- Examination reveals no signs of trauma. Breath sounds are clear and equal with assisted ventilation via a bag-valve-mask. The patient has been incontinent of urine. The trachea is midline and there is no jugular venous distention noted.
- The cardiac monitor reveals the rhythm below.
- How will you manage this patient?

Lead II

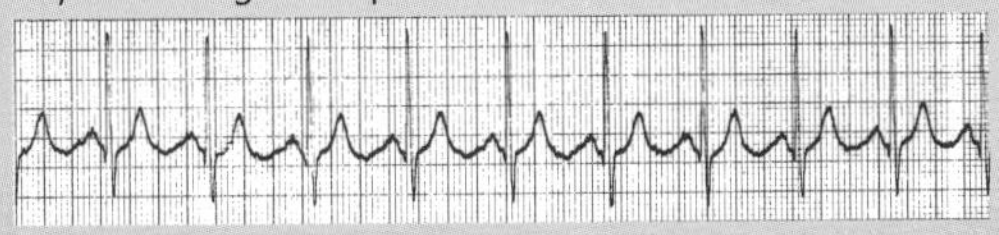

## PUTTING IT ALL TOGETHER

A 79 year old female is complaining of shortness of breath and mid-sternal chest pain radiating to her left arm. She states the pain began yesterday and was tolerable until about 20 minutes ago. On a 1-10 scale, she ranks her pain an 8. The patient states she is nauseated but has not vomited. BP 170/94, respirations 24. The cardiac monitor displays the rhythm below. The patient is allergic to sulfa and underwent back surgery one year ago for which she takes Tylenol #3 as needed.

How will you manage this patient?

Lead II

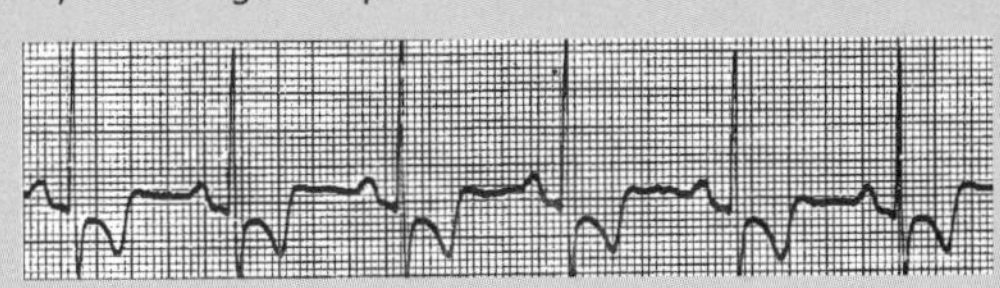

## PUTTING IT ALL TOGETHER

- This patient is a 77 year old male complaining of nonradiating substernal chest "pressure." The patient's pain has been present for 20 minutes and began while watching television. The patient has had no relief of pain from self-administered nitroglycerin x 3 (Nitrostat bottle dated September 1983). On a 1-10 scale, the patient ranks his pain an 8. His blood pressure is 138/64, respiratory rate 20 and non-labored. The physical examination is unremarkable. The patient has a history of angina and duodenal ulcers. Medications include Inderal and Nitrostat.
- An order for atropine 0.5 mg IV bolus over 2 minutes has been received. Do you agree with this order? Why or why not?

Lead II

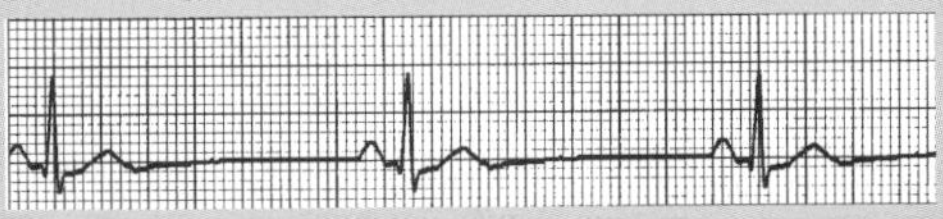

## PUTTING IT ALL TOGETHER

- A 45 year old male is the victim of an electrocution. It appears he was putting up an antenna and struck a live wire while standing on wet grass. The utility company estimates the patient received approximately 7200 volts.
- The patient is moaning and combative. Examination of the head is unremarkable. Pupils are equal and reactive to light. Examination of the chest reveals no sign of injury. Breath sounds are clear and equal bilaterally with a respiratory rate of 28. The abdomen is soft and no wounds are noted. The pelvis is intact. Examination of the back reveals second degree burns to the lumbar area of the spine. Examination of the extremities reveal possible exit wounds and 3rd degree burns to the left medial knee, calf and toes and the right knee.
- Blood pressure is 102/80. The cardiac monitor reveals a sinus tachycardia at 150 beats/minute without ectopy. The patient's skin is cool and wet.
- How will you manage this patient?

## PUTTING IT ALL TOGETHER

- It is 9:00 a.m. when a 59 year old male is brought to the Emergency Department complaining of weakness. The patient states he vomited blood last evening at approximately 8:00 p.m. and then again this morning at 8:00 a.m. Throughout the night the patient states he had episodes of rectal bleeding.
- Physical examination reveals the pupils to be equal and reactive to light. Lungs are clear bilaterally. The abdomen is soft and the patient denies tenderness on palpation. The pelvis is intact. Examination of the extremities is unremarkable.
- Initial vital signs are as follows: BP 80/60, pulse 116 (weak but regular), respirations 16-20. The skin is warm, dry and pale. The cardiac monitor shows a sinus tachycardia without ectopy.
- The patient has a history of duodenal ulcers, cirrhosis of the liver and GI bleeding. His medications include Lasix, Lorazepam, Flurazepam and Chlordiazepoxide.
- How will you manage this patient?

## PUTTING IT ALL TOGETHER

- A 69 year old male states he was golfing when he had a sudden onset of left-sided chest pain and shortness of breath. He states there is no change in his pain on deep inspiration. On a 1-10 scale, he ranks his pain a 6-7.
- The patient is awake and alert. Breath sounds are clear bilaterally with a respiratory rate of 20-22 breaths/minute. Examination of the abdomen, pelvis and extremities are unremarkable. The patient's skin is cool and moist.
- The patient has a history of gout and an "irregular heart beat" and takes Zyloprim.
- Initial vital signs are: BP 70/40, R 20. The cardiac monitor shows atrial fibrillation with a ventricular response of 90-120.
- How will you manage this patient?

## PUTTING IT ALL TOGETHER

- It is 12 noon when a 91 year old female arrives in the Emergency Department complaining of "squeezing" substernal chest pain with radiation to her left arm. The patient states the pain began early this morning. Her husband states he gave her a nitroglycerin tablet at 4 a.m., 7 a.m., 9 a.m. and 10 a.m. with no relief of pain.
- Physical examination reveals the pupils to be equal and reactive to light. The lungs are clear bilaterally with a respiratory rate of 20 per minute. The abdomen is soft and nontender with no distention noted. No pedal edema is noted. The patient's skin is cool, pale and moist. Initial vital signs reveal a blood pressure of 72/40 and a weak, irregular pulse.
- The patient has a hiatal hernia and had a heart attack 1 year ago. Medications include: Nitroglycerin, Tenormin, Metoclopramide, Cardene and Clonidine.
- Describe your management of this patient.

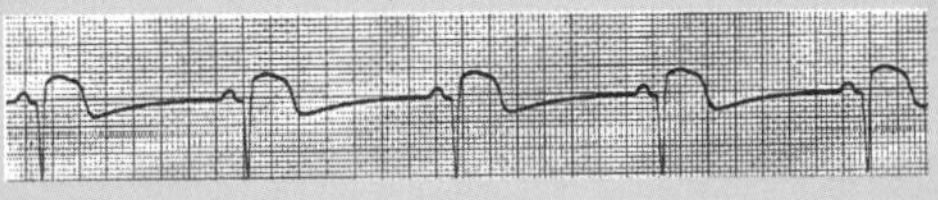

Lead II

## PUTTING IT ALL TOGETHER

- A 55 year old female arrived in the Emergency Department complaining of severe chest pain and difficulty breathing. Her initial blood pressure was 54/P, respirations 8 per minute. The cardiac monitor displayed a narrow-QRS tachycardia at 190 beats/minute. Oxygen therapy was initiated and IV line established. You delivered a synchronized countershock with 50 joules and now note the following rhythm on the cardiac monitor.
- The leads are in place and the patient is now pulseless and apneic. How should you proceed in the management of this patient?

Lead II

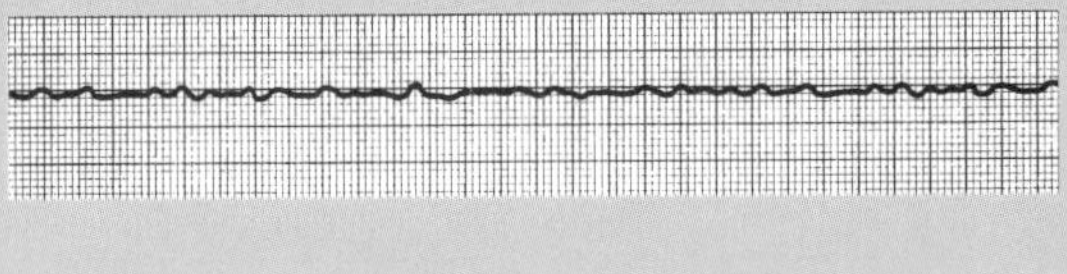

## PUTTING IT ALL TOGETHER

- A sinus rhythm with inverted T waves is shown on the monitor.
- Administer oxygen and establish IV access.
- Administer medications for relief of pain.
- Administer aspirin (if not contraindicated) and evaluate the patient for possible thrombolytic therapy.

## PUTTING IT ALL TOGETHER

- Despite the presence of a sinus rhythm on the cardiac monitor, the patient is pulseless. This situation is termed Pulseless Electrical Activity (PEA).
- Remove the nitropatch on the left upper chest, continue CPR, hyperventilate the patient and prepare the necessary equipment for endotracheal intubation. Confirm placement of the endotracheal tube.
- Establish a large bore IV line of normal saline or lactated Ringer's solution and administer a 500 ml fluid challenge.
- Consider the possible causes of the situation at hand (MATCHx4ED).
  - Myocardial infarction (massive), Acidosis, Tension pneumothorax, Cardiac tamponade, Hypovolemia (most common cause), Hypoxia, Hypothermia, Hyperkalemia, Embolism (massive pulmonary), Drug overdose (cyclic antidepressants, digitalis, beta-blockers, calcium channel blockers)
- If no specific treatable cause can be determined:
  - Administer epinephrine 1 mg IV bolus every 3-5 minutes

## PUTTING IT ALL TOGETHER

- Cervical spine precautions
- Administer oxygen and establish IV access.
  - Rapid IV fluid administration is indicated to:
    - counteract shock
    - correct ongoing fluid losses
    - maintain a diuresis to avoid renal shutdown due to myoglobinuria
- Treat the burns - consult with burn specialist as needed
- Pulse oximetry, continuous ECG monitoring; obtain 12-lead ECG
- Roentgenograms of the cervical spine, chest and extremities
- Laboratory studies including urine analysis, urine myoglobin, CBC, ABGs, SMAC.

## PUTTING IT ALL TOGETHER

- Administer oxygen and establish an IV.
- If the patient's chest pain persists despite oxygen administration, administer medication for pain relief. Sublingual nitroglycerin should be considered since the patient's prescription bottle was dated 10 years ago. If his pain persists despite the administration of nitroglycerin (sublingual nitroglycerin may be administered every 5 minutes to a maximum of 3 doses if needed), administer morphine.
- The cardiac monitor displays a sinus bradycardia. The question that must be asked is: Is the bradycardia the cause of this patient's signs and symptoms? The patient's blood pressure is 138/64, there are no signs of CHF, ventricular ectopy or hypoperfusion. The patient's bradycardia may be a result of the Inderal (a beta-blocker) the patient is taking.
  - If signs and symptoms indicating the use of atropine were present, atropine should be administered RAPID IV bolus (not over 2 minutes). Administration of atropine in doses of less than 0.5 mg increments may further slow the heart rate.

## PUTTING IT ALL TOGETHER

- Administer oxygen and establish IV access.
- This patient is hypotensive and the cardiac monitor shows atrial fibrillation at 90-120 beats/minute. The key question that should be asked is: Is this a rate problem, a pump problem, or a volume problem?
- The patient's breath sounds are clear. Administer a 200-250 ml fluid challenge and reevaluate the patient's condition.
  - This patient's chest pain and shortness of breath resolved after 7-8 minutes of oxygen therapy.
  - Administration of a 200 ml fluid challenge resulted in a change in the patient's blood pressure to 90/70. Additional fluids were ordered. After infusion of 750 ml of normal saline, the patient's blood pressure was 110/74.

## PUTTING IT ALL TOGETHER

- This patient is hypotensive. The key question to ask is: Are the patient's signs and symptoms due to a rate problem, pump problem, or volume problem? Given the patient's history of the present illness, we assume a volume problem exists.
- Administer oxygen, establish two large-bore IV's of normal saline or lactated Ringer's solution and administer a fluid challenge (a fluid challenge of 10-20 ml/kg may be ordered and the frequency of additional boluses adjusted depending on the patient's response).
- Pulse oximetry, 12-lead ECG, chest roentgenogram
- Obtain laboratory studies including CBC, electrolytes, blood type and cross, urinalysis, ABGs.

## PUTTING IT ALL TOGETHER

- Assure the synchronizer switch is off.
- Immediately defibrillate with 200 joules.
- Reassess.

## PUTTING IT ALL TOGETHER

- The rhythm shown is a sinus bradycardia with elevated ST segments.
- Administer oxygen and establish IV access.
- The patient is hypotensive. The key question is: Are the patient's signs and symptoms due to a rate problem, pump problem or volume problem?
- A fluid challenge of 200-250 ml of normal saline may be ordered to rule out hypovolemia. If this therapy proves unsuccessful, administer 0.5-1.0 mg of atropine RAPID IV bolus and reassess.
  - Atropine may be repeated every 3-5 minutes as necessary to a maximum of 2-3 mg.
- If atropine administration does not produce a satisfactory response, prepare for transcutaneous pacing.

## PUTTING IT ALL TOGETHER

- You are a Paramedic called to the scene of an assault. On arrival police officers are performing CPR on a 33 year old male lying supine in front of a trailer. They state the patient was struck in the chest with a shovel an unknown number of times. You have confirmed the patient is unresponsive, pulseless and apneic.
- An oropharyngeal airway is inserted and the patient ventilated with 100% oxygen. Physical examination reveals significant bruising, marked deformity and crepitus of the anterior chest. The head is intact with no signs of trauma noted. The abdomen is soft and no distention is noted. The pelvis is intact and the extremities show no signs of trauma.
- The cardiac monitor reveals the rhythm below. Describe your management of this patient.

Lead II

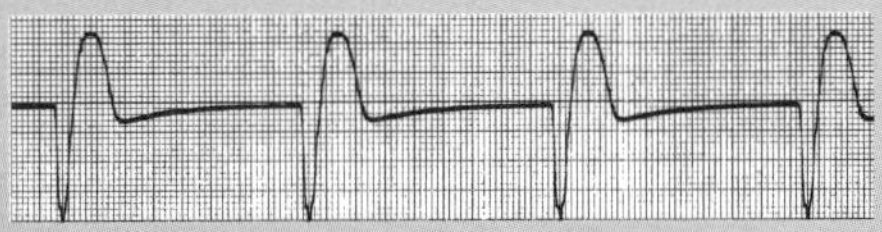

## PUTTING IT ALL TOGETHER

- A 73 year old patient is complaining of a sudden onset of lightheadedness and palpitations. She denies chest pain but is extremely anxious. The cardiac monitor shows atrial fibrillation with a ventricular response of 160-210 beats per minute.
- The patient's blood pressure is 122/70, respirations 16. Breath sounds are clear.
- How will you manage this patient?

## PUTTING IT ALL TOGETHER

- It is a hot July day. You are a Paramedic called to the scene of an "unconscious male." On arrival you find a 23 year old male unconscious and unresponsive to a sternal rub lying on the grass near a swimming pool. Bystanders state the patient was swimming and went under the water for approximately 1-2 minutes. When they realized the patient hadn't surfaced for some time, they went in and got him and then called 911. These bystanders initiated rescue breathing until the patient began breathing on his own. They state the patient did not suffer any trauma prior to the incident and indicate the patient has been drinking heavily today.
- The patient is lying on his left side with a respiratory rate of 2-4 breaths per minute. A pulse is present at 80 beats/minute and the blood pressure is 118/70. The cardiac monitor displays a sinus rhythm at 80 without ectopy.
- What should be done for the patient at this time?
- Should this patient be transported to a medical facility?

## PUTTING IT ALL TOGETHER

- A 62 year old male is complaining of a sudden onset of chest pain and difficulty breathing. The cardiac rhythm reveals the rhythm below.
- The patient's blood pressure is 76/54 and respirations are 14-16 per minute. Breath sounds are clear. The patient has no significant past medical history.
- How will you manage this patient?

Lead II

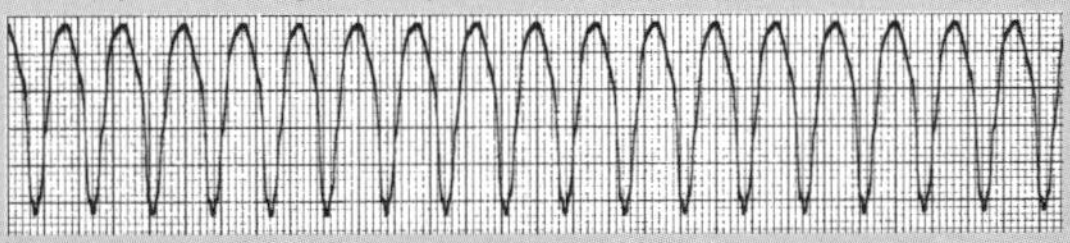

## PUTTING IT ALL TOGETHER

An 86 year old female is complaining of nausea and "heaviness" in her chest. She states she was awakened from sleep with nausea, sweating and severe chest pain. The pain has been present and persistent for 1 1/2 hours. She has a past medical history of an irregular heart rate and CHF for which she takes Theodur, Lanoxin, Lasix and Roxicet. Breath sounds are clear bilaterally. No edema of the lower extremities is noted. The remainder of the physical exam is unremarkable. BP 152/80, pulse irregular, respirations 20. The cardiac monitor shows a sinus rhythm at 88 with a run of ventricular tachycardia.
How will you manage this patient?

## PUTTING IT ALL TOGETHER

- It is 3:00 a.m. when a 36 year old female, 8 months pregnant, arrives in the Emergency Department complaining of dizziness, severe abdominal pain and vaginal bleeding. She states she was involved in an altercation with her boyfriend and sister about 1 hour ago during which her sister fell on her abdomen. The patient admits to consuming 5-6 bottles of beer since midnight and states she has seen a physician once during her pregnancy.
- Examination reveals a blood pressure of 70/54 while supine, pulse of 120 (sinus tachycardia) and a respiratory rate of 18-22. Breath sounds are clear. The physical examination is unremarkable with the exception of a distended, pregnant abdomen and approximately 200 ml of blood noted on the patient's clothing. Regular fetal heart tones at a rate of 140 beats/minute are present on auscultation.
- How will you manage this patient?

## PUTTING IT ALL TOGETHER

- An 82 year old male is brought to your facility by Paramedics unable to move his left side. The patient's wife states the patient was lying in bed and was unable to get up.
- The patient is able to follow commands and states his name when questioned. A left-sided facial droop is noted with a fixed gaze to the right. Breath sounds are clear but diminished in the lower lobes. The abdomen is soft and non-tender, no masses are palpated. The pelvis is intact with incontinence of urine noted. The patient has a strong right-sided grip with no response on the left. Examination of the back is unremarkable.
- The cardiac monitor shows a sinus rhythm without ectopy. Initial vital signs reveal a blood pressure of 150/84, pulse 80 (strong and regular), respirations 20. The skin is warm and dry.
- The patient has a history of carotid artery surgery and hypertension. Medications include Procardia, Lanoxin, Ecotrin, Hydrochlorothiazide and Propranolol.
- Describe your management of this patient.

## PUTTING IT ALL TOGETHER

Three primary mechanisms regulate the hydrogen ion concentration in the body. Name them, beginning with the most rapidly acting mechanism.

## PUTTING IT ALL TOGETHER

- Administer oxygen and establish IV access.
- The objective in the management of this patient will be to slow the ventricular rate. Medications which may be considered are:
  - Beta-blockers (Esmolol, Propranolol, Metoprolol)
  - Calcium channel blockers (Diltiazem, Verapamil)
  - Digoxin

## PUTTING IT ALL TOGETHER

- Despite the presence of an idioventricular rhythm on the cardiac monitor, the patient is pulseless. This situation is termed Pulseless Electrical Activity (PEA).
- Continue CPR, hyperventilate the patient and prepare the necessary equipment for endotracheal intubation. Confirm placement of the endotracheal tube. Establish two large bore IV lines of normal saline or lactated Ringer's solution and administer a 500 ml fluid challenge.
- Consider the possible causes of the situation at hand (MATCHx4ED).
  - Myocardial infarction (massive), Acidosis, Tension pneumothorax, Cardiac tamponade, Hypovolemia (most common cause), Hypoxia, Hypothermia, Hyperkalemia, Embolism (massive pulmonary), Drug overdose (cyclic anti-depressants, digitalis, beta-blockers, calcium channel blockers)
- If no specific treatable cause can be determined:
  - Administer epinephrine 1 mg IV bolus every 3-5 minutes. The rhythm shown is a bradycardia. Administer atropine 1 mg IV bolus every 3-5 minutes to a maximum of 3 mg.

## PUTTING IT ALL TOGETHER

- This patient is unstable (chest pain, hypotension).
- Wide-QRS tachycardias associated with pulselessness, shock or CHF are treated as if the rhythm is ventricular tachycardia.
- Administer oxygen and establish IV access.
- Administer lidocaine if it is immediately available and administration will not delay countershock.
- Administer sedation and deliver an unsynchronized countershock with 100, 200, 300, and 360 joules as needed
- Unsynchronized countershocks are administered to the patient in VT who is hypotensive, unresponsive or in the presence of pulmonary edema (October 1992 JAMA, p 2212).

## PUTTING IT ALL TOGETHER

- Administer 100% oxygen and assist ventilations with a bag-valve-mask device.
- Establish IV access and provide supportive care as needed.
- Yes, this patient should be transported to a medical facility. "Every submersion victim, even one who requires only minimal resuscitation and regains consciousness at the scene, should be transferred to a medical facility for follow-up care."
  - Emergency Cardiac Care Committee and Subcommittees, American Heart Association. Guidelines for cardiopulmonary resuscitation and emergency cardiac care. JAMA 268:2246, 1992.

## PUTTING IT ALL TOGETHER

- This patient is at risk for, or may be experiencing, abruptio placenta.
- Administer high flow oxygen and establish IV access with two large bore IVs of normal saline or lactated Ringer's solution.
- Turn the patient on her left side in an effort to move the weight of the gravid uterus off the vena cava and abdominal aorta.
- Administer a fluid challenge of 20 ml/kg.
- Evaluate fetal heart tones.
- Pulse oximetry, lab studies, ultrasound of the abdomen.
- Transfer to the obstetrical unit for definitive care as soon as possible.

## PUTTING IT ALL TOGETHER

- Administer oxygen, establish IV access.
- Administer medication for pain relief.
- Administer aspirin (if not contraindicated).
- Determine if the patient is a candidate for thrombolytic therapy (age 86 years).
- If the ventricular ectopy persists despite oxygen administration and medications for relief of pain, administer lidocaine.
  - Initial bolus 1-1.5 mg/kg repeated as needed with 1/2 this dose (0.5-0.75 mg/kg) every 5 minutes. The maintenance infusion rate should be reduced by 1/2 that normally administered due to the patient's age.

## PUTTING IT ALL TOGETHER

- The buffer system (most rapid)
- The respiratory system
- The renal system

## PUTTING IT ALL TOGETHER

- Administer oxygen.
- Establish IV access with normal saline and infuse at 30 ml/hour.
- Pulse oximetry, continuous ECG monitoring, obtain 12-lead ECG
- Portable chest roentgenogram
- Laboratory studies including: electrolytes, glucose, CBC and coagulation studies, ABGs
- Assess Glasgow Coma Scale
- Neuro consult
- CT of the brain without contrast.

## PUTTING IT ALL TOGETHER

- You are a Paramedic called for an "ill man". On arrival, you find a 76 year old male cyanotic, pulseless and apneic. As you direct your crew to begin CPR the patient's wife tells you the patient was seen in the Emergency Department yesterday for chest pain and released. She also states the patient started "feeling sick" this morning and then collapsed in front of her about 10 minutes ago. The patient has a congenital heart defect and takes Lanoxin. He is allergic to Penicillin.
- A quick-look reveals VF. Defibrillation is performed with 200, 300 and 360 joules without change in the patient's rhythm or condition. The patient is successfully intubated and is being ventilated with 100% oxygen via a bag-valve device and an IV of normal saline is established.
- The cardiac monitor now displays the rhythm below. How should you proceed?

Lead II

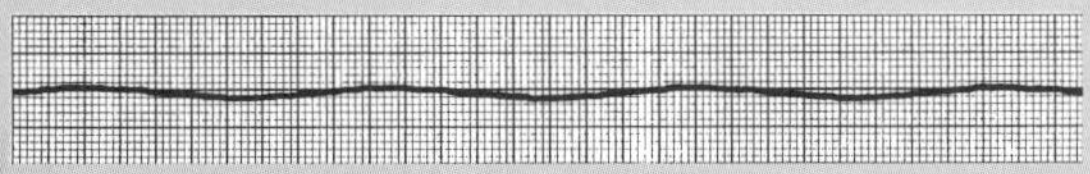

## PUTTING IT ALL TOGETHER

- Resuscitation efforts are in progress for an 84 year old female in cardiac arrest. The monitor displays ventricular fibrillation. Initial defibrillation attempts have proven unsuccessful. The patient has been intubated and an IV line has been established. 1.0 mg of epinephrine was administered and the patient defibrillated with 360J. A lidocaine bolus of 1.5 mg/kg and a subsequent defibrillation with 360J has proven unsuccessful. The patient's condition is unchanged and the monitor reveals VF.
- A lidocaine bolus has been administered, should you now establish a lidocaine drip?

## PUTTING IT ALL TOGETHER

Why is procainamide less desirable than adenosine in the management of the stable patient with a wide-complex tachycardia of uncertain origin?

## PUTTING IT ALL TOGETHER

What is the "door-to-drug" interval?

## PUTTING IT ALL TOGETHER

- It is 7:30 p.m. when a 70 year old female arrives in the Emergency Department complaining of a sudden onset of chest pain that began at 5 p.m. while watching television. At 6 p.m. the patient took one aspirin with no relief of pain. The patient states she has never had this pain before. The pain radiates to her left arm, neck and jaw and left shoulder. She denies nausea or shortness of breath. On a 1-10 scale, the patient ranks her pain an 8.
- Her blood pressure is 146/82, pulse 98 and regular (sinus rhythm), respiratory rate 24 and nonlabored. Her skin is warm and dry.
- How will you manage this patient?

## PUTTING IT ALL TOGETHER

- An 86 year old, 75 kg, male is pulseless and apneic. The cardiac monitor displays the rhythm below.
- Defibrillation with 200, 300 and 360 joules has resulted in no change in the rhythm. CPR has been resumed and the patient has been successfully intubated, however, repeated attempts to establish an IV have proven futile.
- How will you proceed?

Lead II

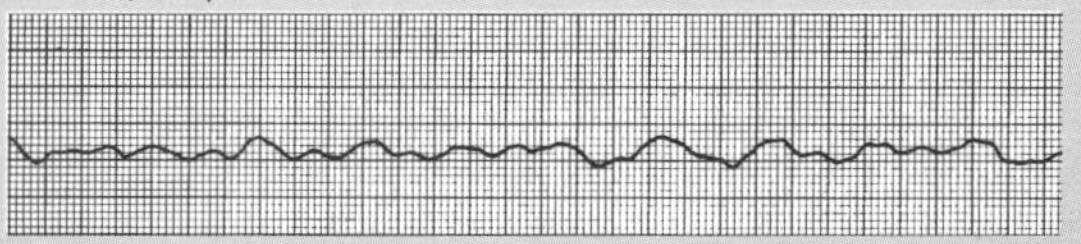

## PUTTING IT ALL TOGETHER

Name four tasks that should be assigned by the team leader at the start of a resuscitation effort.

## PUTTING IT ALL TOGETHER

Name two possible complications of CPR.

## PUTTING IT ALL TOGETHER

- No. Only bolus therapy should be used in cardiac arrest.
- Upon return of spontaneous circulation, an infusion of 2-4 mg/minute should be started.
    - Upon return of spontaneous circulation, lidocaine should NOT be administered for a ventricular escape rhythm.

## PUTTING IT ALL TOGETHER

- Confirm the rhythm in another lead. If confirmed as asystole:
    - Continue CPR.
    - Consider possible causes of the arrest (hypoxia, hypokalemia, hyperkalemia, hypothermia, preexisting acidosis, drug overdose).
    - Consider transcutaneous pacing
    - Administer 1 mg (1:10,000) epinephrine IV bolus. Reassess. This may be repeated every 3-5 minutes or alternative dosing regimens may be administered after administration of the first bolus.
    - If no response, administer 1 mg of atropine IV bolus. This may be repeated every 3-5 minutes to a maximum dose of 3 mg.
- Consider termination of efforts if no response to treatment.

## PUTTING IT ALL TOGETHER

- The interval from the patient's arrival in the Emergency Department to the start of delivery of thrombolytic agents has been referred to as the "door-to-drug" interval.
- Emergency Departments should take no more than 30-60 minutes to assess and begin thrombolytic treatment for patients with evidence of coronary thrombosis and no reasons for exclusion.

## PUTTING IT ALL TOGETHER

Procainamide has a greater potential for lowering blood pressure and takes longer to work.

## PUTTING IT ALL TOGETHER

- Continue attempts to establish IV access.
- Administer epinephrine via the endotracheal tube.
    - The endotracheal dose is 2-2.5 times the IV dose. Since the initial IV bolus is 1 mg, administer 2 or 2.5 mg (use the 1:1000 concentration and dilute with normal saline for a total volume of 10 ml).
- Defibrillate with 360 joules and reassess.
- If no change, resume CPR.
- Administer lidocaine via the endotracheal tube.
    - The endotracheal dose is 2-2.5 times the IV dose. Since the initial IV bolus is 1 or 1.5 mg/kg, administer 2 or 3 mg/kg and dilute as needed for a total volume of 10 ml.

## PUTTING IT ALL TOGETHER

- Administer oxygen and establish IV access.
- Administer sublingual nitroglycerin and repeat if needed every 5 minutes to a maximum dose of 3 tablets.
- If no relief of pain with nitroglycerin, administer morphine 1-3 mg IV bolus every 5 minutes titrated to pain relief.
- The patient has already taken an aspirin prior to her arrival in the Emergency Department so additional therapy is not needed at this time.
- If evidence of coronary thrombosis present, evaluate the patient for possible thrombolytic therapy.

## PUTTING IT ALL TOGETHER

Possible complications of CPR include:

- Aspiration
- Liver laceration
- Gastric rupture
- Pulmonary contusion
- Mediastinal hemorrhage
- Spleen laceration/rupture
- Rib and/or sternal fractures
    - Pneumothorax, flail chest, pericardial tamponade

## PUTTING IT ALL TOGETHER

- Airway and intubation
- Chest compressions
- Monitoring and defibrillation
- Intravenous access

## PUTTING IT ALL TOGETHER

A 27 year old female, 8 1/2 months pregnant, has suffered a traumatic cardiac arrest.

Explain why displacement of the uterus to the left during resuscitation efforts is important.

## PUTTING IT ALL TOGETHER

Name two advantages of mechanical chest compressors.

## PUTTING IT ALL TOGETHER

- A 77 year old male is complaining of chest pain radiating down his left arm that has been present for the past 1 1/2 hours and rates his pain a 10 on a 1-10 scale. The patient has taken 6 nitroglycerin tablets with no relief of pain. His BP is 170/72, R 18. Breath sounds are clear.
- The patient's past medical history is significant for an angioplasty 1 month ago, coronary bypass surgery 5 years ago, an artificial valve and a history of hypertension. He takes Nitroglycerin, Coumadin, Digitalis, Procardia and Vicodin. The patient is allergic to aspirin.
- How will you manage this patient?

Lead II

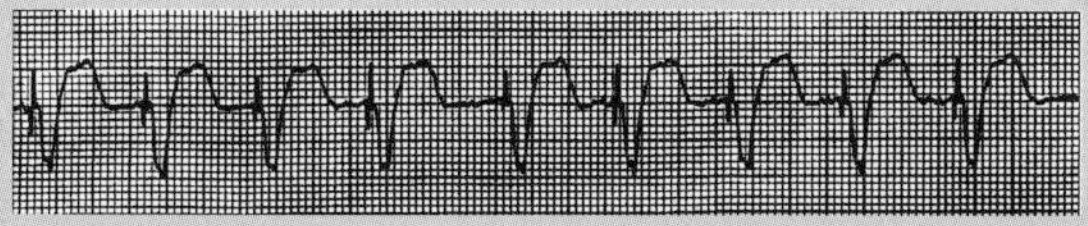

## PUTTING IT ALL TOGETHER

- An 18 year old victim of a drive-by shooting is brought to your facility by his family. Examination reveals the patient to be responsive only to painful stimuli with a blood pressure of 60/40, labored respirations at 28 per minute, and a pulse rate of 140 (sinus tachycardia).
- A single gunshot wound is found on the right side of the chest in the fourth intercostal space, mid-axillary line. Breath sounds are absent on the right and diminished on the left. The right side of the chest is hyperresonant to percussion.
- How will you manage this patient?

## PUTTING IT ALL TOGETHER

Bradycardias and tachycardias may produce serious signs and symptoms.

Name four signs and symptoms that, if present, would cause you to consider the patient "unstable."

## PUTTING IT ALL TOGETHER

- A 47 year old male has arrived in the Emergency Department complaining of severe chest pain present for the past 3 hours. He has a history of "heart problems" and ulcers. As you administer oxygen and initiate an IV, the patient arrests. The cardiac monitor reveals ventricular fibrillation.
- After 15 minutes, your efforts in resuscitating this patient have resulted in a palpable pulse. The patient has been intubated. The monitor now shows a complete (third-degree) AV block with a wide-QRS at a rate of 32 beats/minute. The blood pressure is 64/40 and there are no spontaneous respirations.
- How will you manage this patient?

## PUTTING IT ALL TOGETHER

When is use of the pneumatic antishock garment (PASG) indicated?

## PUTTING IT ALL TOGETHER

- A 79 year old female is complaining of severe chest pain radiating to both arms. The patient states her pain began 20 minutes ago during a meeting. On a 1-10 scale, she ranks her pain a 9 and states her arms are numb.
- The cardiac monitor reveals the rhythm below. Her blood pressure is 142/84, respiratory rate 24. Breath sounds are clear.
- The patient has a history of a CVA 4 years ago and takes Lanoxin and Tenormin.
- How will you manage this patient?

Lead II

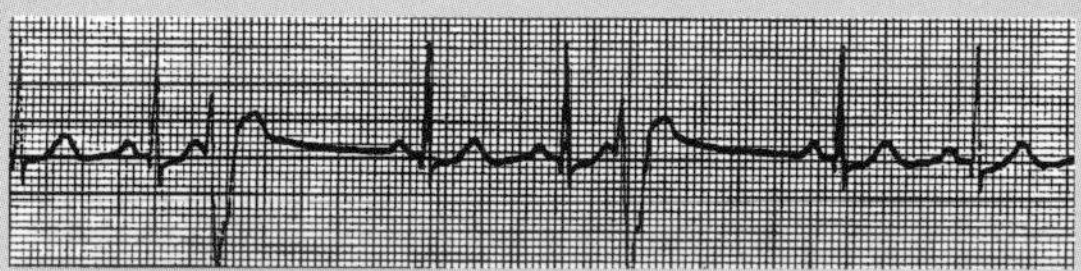

## PUTTING IT ALL TOGETHER

Mechanical chest compressors:

- eliminate rescuer fatigue
- standardize the technique of CPR
- free trained persons to participate in the delivery of ACLS when there is a limited number of rescuers
- assure adequacy of compressions when a patient requires continued resuscitation during transportation.

## PUTTING IT ALL TOGETHER

Manual displacement of the uterus to the left side while CPR is in progress is extremely important because compression of the gravid uterus on the abdominal aorta and inferior vena cava markedly reduces uteroplacental blood flow and venous return to the heart.

## PUTTING IT ALL TOGETHER

- This patient is exhibiting signs and symptoms of a tension pneumothorax.
- Perform a needle thoracostomy.
  - Insert a large bore (14 gauge) needle into the second intercostal space, midclavicular line.
- Administer oxygen, establish IV access.
- Pulse oximetry, 12-lead ECG, portable chest and abdominal roentgenograms, lab studies.
- Surgical evaluation as soon as possible.
  - Performance of a needle thoracostomy resulted in an escape of air (relief of the tension pneumothorax). Repeat vitals after the needle thoracostomy revealed the patient's blood pressure to be 118/70, pulse 90, respiratory rate 18.

## PUTTING IT ALL TOGETHER

- The rhythm shown is a ventricular paced rhythm at 80.
- Administer oxygen and establish IV access.
- Initiate pulse oximetry, obtain a 12-lead ECG, portable chest roentgenogram, lab studies.
- Administer morphine 1-3 mg (2 mg increments) every 5 minutes titrated to pain relief.
- Administration of 6 mg of morphine resulted in relief of pain.

## PUTTING IT ALL TOGETHER

- Continue ventilating the patient with 100% oxygen with a bag-valve device until a ventilator is available.
- Initiate transcutaneous pacing and note the patient's response to this intervention (blood pressure, pulse, etc.).
- Although the patient was in VF, lidocaine should NOT be administered. The wide-QRS indicates the presence of a ventricular escape rhythm and administration of lidocaine in this situation may be lethal.
- Order chest roentgenogram, lab studies.
- Reassess frequently.

## PUTTING IT ALL TOGETHER

- Signs of shock
- Shortness of breath
- Persistent chest pain
- Pulmonary congestion
- Congestive heart failure
- Decreased blood pressure
- Acute myocardial infarction
- Decreased level of consciousness

## PUTTING IT ALL TOGETHER

- Administer oxygen and establish IV access.
- Administer medications for pain relief (nitroglycerin, morphine).
- Administer aspirin if no reason for exclusion.
- Order lab work to include potassium and magnesium levels.
- Due to the presence of frequent R on T PVCs, administer lidocaine IV bolus and prepare a continuous lidocaine infusion.
  - Due to the patient's age, the infusion rate should be 1/2 that normally administered.

## PUTTING IT ALL TOGETHER

Currently, the primary use of the pneumatic antishock garment (MAST suit) is for hypovolemic shock secondary to bleeding in the lower half of the body.

## PUTTING IT ALL TOGETHER

What is the compression rate for two-rescuer adult CPR?

## PUTTING IT ALL TOGETHER

- A 46 year old male is complaining of a sudden onset of substernal chest pain radiating to his left arm and lower jaw. His pain began approximately 25 minutes ago at rest and has been steadily increasing in intensity. On a 1-10 scale, the patient rates his pain a 10. The patient states he vomited undigested food about 20 minutes ago and is nauseated. He has no significant past medical history.
- His blood pressure is 62/44. Respiratory rate is 20-24 per minute. His skin is cool, clammy and pale. The cardiac monitor reveals a complete (third-degree) AV block with a narrow-QRS and a ventricular response of 48 beats/minute and elevated ST segments.
- How will you manage this patient?

## PUTTING IT ALL TOGETHER

- It is 7:00 a.m. when Paramedics are called to the home of a 49 year old male complaining of difficulty breathing and epigastric pain. His BP is 64/P, respiratory rate 30 and shallow, and the skin is warm, pale and moist. Breath sounds are clear. The patient denies chest pain. The abdomen is tender in the epigastric region on palpation. Femoral pulses are equal and a dressing located in the right inguinal region is dry. Examination of the lower extremities reveals no significant findings.
- The patient's past medical history is significant for a right inguinal hernia operation yesterday performed on an out-patient basis. His history is otherwise negative. The patient states he took 2 extra-strength Tylenol at 3 a.m. with no relief of pain. A second set of vital signs reveals: BP 62/30, pulse 110 (sinus tach), R 24.
- What should be done at this point?

## PUTTING IT ALL TOGETHER

When should invasive (open-chest) CPR be considered?

## PUTTING IT ALL TOGETHER

Name two forms of acid produced during aerobic metabolism.

## PUTTING IT ALL TOGETHER

- A 54 year old male is complaining of retrosternal chest pain and numbness in both arms. The patient appears to be in acute distress and ranks his pain an 8 on a 1-10 scale. He has taken two Tylenol tablets since the pain began approximately 2 hours ago without relief.
- Examination reveals a blood pressure of 80/60 and a respiratory rate of 14. The cardiac monitor shows a sinus rhythm at 78 without ectopy. Breath sounds are clear and the remainder of the physical examination is unremarkable.
- The patient's past medical history is significant for a myocardial infarction 3 years ago. The patient takes no medications regularly and has no known allergies.
- You are asked to administer 0.4 mg of nitroglycerin sublingually.
- Do you agree with this order? Why or why not?

## PUTTING IT ALL TOGETHER

Name two advantages of the automatic chest compressor (cardiac thumper).

## PUTTING IT ALL TOGETHER

- A 55 year old male is complaining of substernal, nonradiating chest pain that he describes as a "squeezing" sensation. He states the pain started after a family fight and has been present for 2 hours.
- Blood pressure is 160/90, respirations 18. Breath sounds are clear. The cardiac monitor reveals a sinus tachycardia at 138 beats per minute.
- The patient has a history of high blood pressure, "heart problems" and diabetes for which he takes Capoten, Diabeta, and Prednisone.
- How will you manage this patient?

## PUTTING IT ALL TOGETHER

- Administer oxygen and establish IV access.
- Administer atropine 0.5-1.0 mg IV every 3-5 minutes to a maximum dose of 2-3 mg. Prepare for transcutaneous pacing.
- Administration of medications for pain relief should be withheld until the patient's systolic blood pressure is >100 mm Hg systolic.
- Administer aspirin if no reason for exclusion.

## PUTTING IT ALL TOGETHER

The compression rate for two-rescuer adult CPR is 80-100 per minute.

## PUTTING IT ALL TOGETHER

- Penetrating chest trauma
- Blunt trauma with cardiac arrest
- Penetrating abdominal trauma with deterioration and cardiac arrest
- Chest deformity where closed-chest CPR is not effective
- Consider in cardiac arrest due to:
  - hypothermia
  - pulmonary embolism
  - pericardial tamponade
  - abdominal hemorrhage

## PUTTING IT ALL TOGETHER

- Administer oxygen and establish IV access (preferably two large-bore IVs) with normal saline or Ringer's lactate.
- The question to be asked is, "Is this a rate problem, a pump problem or a volume problem"? Based on the patient's history and presenting signs and symptoms, possibilities include abdominal bleeding, pulmonary embolism, myocardial infarction.
- Administer a fluid challenge of 10-20 ml/kg and reevaluate.
  - Despite the administration of 4 liters of normal saline, the patient's blood pressure remained 64/P. Lab studies revealed a hemoglobin of 7 and a hematocrit of 27. The patient was taken to the operating room for resolution of post-operative hemorrhage.

## PUTTING IT ALL TOGETHER

- Administer oxygen and establish IV access.
- Administer aspirin if no reason for exclusion.
- The patient's blood pressure is 80/60. Breath sounds are clear. Administer a 200-250 ml fluid challenge and reassess the patient's blood pressure.
- Medications for pain relief should be withheld until the patient's systolic blood pressure is > 100 mm Hg.
  - Administration of a 250 ml fluid challenge of normal saline resulted in a systolic BP of 110/70. Sublingual nitroglycerin was administered x 2 without relief of pain. BP 108/70. After 2 mg of morphine IV bolus, the patient stated his pain was a "6". BP 104/70. An additional 2 mg of morphine resolved his chest pain. BP 118/70.
- Evaluate the patient for possible thrombolytic therapy.

## PUTTING IT ALL TOGETHER

Cellular metabolism produces acid. The forms of acid produced during aerobic (in the presence of oxygen) metabolism are:

- Carbon dioxide (excreted by the lungs)
- Metabolic acids
- Lactic acid (the result of the metabolism of fats, acids and carbohydrates)
- Inorganic phosphoric and sulfuric acids.

## PUTTING IT ALL TOGETHER

- Administer oxygen and establish IV access.
- Administer medication for relief of chest pain: nitroglycerin, morphine if no relief from nitroglycerin therapy.
- Administer aspirin (if no reason for exclusion).
- If evidence of coronary thrombosis is evident, evaluate the patient for possible thrombolytic therapy.

## PUTTING IT ALL TOGETHER

- Does not require electrical power (powered by 100% oxygen gas)
- Compressions, ventilations can be adjusted as necessary
- Eliminates variables such as operator technique and rescuer fatigue
- Acceptable ECG can be recorded with compressor in operation
- Patient can be defibrillated or transported without interrupting CPR
- Hemodynamics produced are comparable to those produced during standard manual CPR.

## PUTTING IT ALL TOGETHER

It is essential to frequently assess responses to therapy during a resuscitation effort.

Name three responses that should be frequently evaluated.

## PUTTING IT ALL TOGETHER

- A 60 year old female has suffered a cardiac arrest. The cardiac monitor reveals ventricular fibrillation. You immediately defibrillated the patient with 200 joules which resulted in conversion to a sinus rhythm without ectopy. A pulse is palpable. There are no spontaneous respirations and the blood pressure is 88/60 at this time.
- The patient is successfully intubated and is being ventilated with a bag-valve device. An IV line is established. As you prepare to transfer the patient to the CCU, the patient suddenly deteriorates. The monitor reveals ventricular fibrillation and examination confirms the patient to be pulseless and apneic.
- How should you proceed?

## PUTTING IT ALL TOGETHER

- An 86 year old female is complaining of difficulty breathing which has been present for the past 30 minutes.
- The patient is extremely anxious, speaking in one-word sentences and is in obvious distress. The patient's blood pressure is 184/100, pulse 124 (sinus tach), respiratory rate 32 and labored. The skin is cool and moist. Nasal flaring and accessory muscle usage is evident and jugular venous distention is noted. Auscultation of the chest reveals bilateral crackles. Examination of the extremities reveals no pedal edema.
- The patient has a past medical history of a stroke in June 1991 and peptic ulcers. Medications include Zantac.
- Describe your management of this patient.

## PUTTING IT ALL TOGETHER

Name three reasons for critical incident debriefing.

## PUTTING IT ALL TOGETHER

A 67 year old male is found unresponsive, pulseless and apneic. The cardiac monitor reveals asystole.

Name four possible causes of this condition that should be considered in the management of this patient.

## PUTTING IT ALL TOGETHER

A 54 year old male has arrived in the Emergency Department complaining of crushing chest pain present for the past hour. On a 1-10 scale he rates his pain a 9. His blood pressure is 148/80, respiratory rate 22. The cardiac monitor displays a sinus rhythm at 64 beats per minute. ST-segment elevation of 2 mm is noted in Leads II and III.

- The physical examination reveals the patient to be alert and oriented. Pupils are equal and reactive to light. Breath sounds are clear. The skin is warm, pink and moist. The abdomen is soft and nontender. Motor and sensory responses are within normal limits. Peripheral pulses are strong and equal bilaterally. The patient has no significant past medical history and takes no medications regularly.
- Oxygen therapy has been initiated and an IV established. Sublingual nitroglycerin has been administered x 3 with no relief of pain. Based on the information provided, is this patient a candidate for thrombolytic therapy?

## PUTTING IT ALL TOGETHER

- A 56 year old male is complaining his "heart is racing." He is disoriented and having difficulty breathing. Examination reveals a blood pressure of 64/P; a weak, rapid carotid pulse and pale, cool skin.
- Your ECG shows a narrow-QRS tachycardia at 220 beats/minute.
- Describe your initial management of this patient.

## PUTTING IT ALL TOGETHER

Postresuscitation management should include performance of a complete examination and review of the chest roentgenogram. Special attention should be paid to possible complications of resuscitation.

Name two possible complications of resuscitation related to the respiratory system.

## PUTTING IT ALL TOGETHER

- If the defibrillator is not immediately available, a precordial thump may be attempted since the arrest was witnessed.
- Initiate CPR.
- The previous defibrillation attempt with 200 joules resulted in successful conversion of the rhythm. Defibrillate again with 200 joules.

## PUTTING IT ALL TOGETHER

- Assess pulses with CPR
- Assess the adequacy of ventilations
- Assess pulses after interventions and/or rhythm change
- Assess breathing with a return of pulse
- Assess blood pressure if a pulse is present
- Consider terminating efforts if no response to resuscitation efforts.

## PUTTING IT ALL TOGETHER

Critical incident debriefing:

- Allows review of critical responsibility
- Facilitates "grief work" and accomplishes resolution
- Provides continuing education or "practice reflections"
- Allows discussion of thoughts, feelings and performance
- Permits expression of anxiety, guilt, anger and other emotions.

## PUTTING IT ALL TOGETHER

- Sit the patient up with the legs dependent.
- Administer high flow oxygen and assist ventilations with a bag-valve device. Have intubation equipment ready and be prepared to intubate.
- Establish IV access.
- Attach the cardiac monitor, pulse oximeter.
- Order 12-lead ECG and portable chest roentgenogram.
- First-line medications in the management of acute pulmonary edema include sublingual nitroglycerin, furosemide (0.5-1.0 mg/kg) IV bolus and morphine (1-3 mg administered in 2 mg increments) IV bolus.

## PUTTING IT ALL TOGETHER

- Based on the information provided, the patient is a candidate for thrombolytic therapy (age < 70, presence of chest pain for at least 30 minutes not relieved by sublingual nitroglycerin, ST-segment elevation of at least 1 mm in two anatomically contiguous leads, symptom onset of 6 hours or less, no evidence of absolute contraindications to thrombolytic therapy).
- Baseline lab studies should be obtained (CBC, platelet count, cardiac enzymes, electrolytes, differential, coagulation studies and type and crossmatch).
- Administer aspirin 150-325 mg.
- A 5000 unit IV bolus of heparin and an infusion of 1000 units/hour is recommended immediately after administration of Alteplase (t-PA, Activase) or Streptokinase to help maintain vessel patency.

## PUTTING IT ALL TOGETHER

Possible causes of asystole that should be considered include (Hx4AD):

- Hypoxia
- Hypokalemia
- Hyperkalemia
- Hypothermia
- Acidosis (preexisting)
- Drug overdose

## PUTTING IT ALL TOGETHER

- Rib fractures
- Pneumothorax
- Hemopneumothorax
- Pericardial tamponade
- Improper endotracheal tube placement

## PUTTING IT ALL TOGETHER

- Administer oxygen and establish IV access.
- This patient is unstable as evidenced by his altered level of consciousness, hypotension, and difficulty breathing.
- Administer sedation and deliver a synchronized countershock with 50 joules.
- Reassess the patient's pulse, rhythm and condition. If necessary, subsequent synchronized countershocks may be delivered with 100, 200, 300 and 360 joules, assessing the patient's pulse, rhythm and clinical condition between shocks.

## PUTTING IT ALL TOGETHER

- A 68 year old male is complaining of substernal chest pain radiating to his jaw, weakness and nausea. His blood pressure is 78/56, respiratory rate 16. Breath sounds are clear. The cardiac monitor reveals a second-degree AV block, type I.
- The maximum dose of atropine has been administered to this patient without success and a pacemaker is not immediately available. What is your next course of action?

## PUTTING IT ALL TOGETHER

What is the recommended compression to ventilation ratio in one-rescuer adult CPR?

## PUTTING IT ALL TOGETHER

What is meant by the term "pseudo-EMD"?

## PUTTING IT ALL TOGETHER

Name five primary roles of ACLS team members in a resuscitation effort.

## PUTTING IT ALL TOGETHER

- A 30 year old male has been involved in a automobile accident. The patient, the unrestrained driver of the vehicle, was travelling at a speed of approximately 50 miles per hour when he lost control of his car and hit a light pole.
- The patient is unresponsive, pulseless and apneic. Breath sounds are clear bilaterally. Bruising is noted in the center of the patient's chest. The skin is pale and cold. The cardiac monitor reveals a sinus tachycardia with occasional PVCs. Crepitus is noted on palpation of the pelvis.
- Describe your initial management of this patient.

## PUTTING IT ALL TOGETHER

- A 64 year old male is complaining of nonradiating retrosternal chest pain and difficulty breathing. The patient stated he was eating breakfast when the pain suddenly began. He rates his pain an "8" on a 1-10 scale.
- Examination reveals a BP of 168/84, respirations 32 and labored. Auscultation of the chest reveals crackles in the lower lobes bilaterally. JVD is present to the angle of the jaw. Pitting pedal edema is present to the ankles. The cardiac monitor displays a sinus tachycardia at 140 per minute.
- The patient has a history of emphysema and takes Lanoxin, Zantac, Lasix and Micro K regularly.
- How will you manage this patient?

## PUTTING IT ALL TOGETHER

Name two immediate goals of postresuscitation care.

## PUTTING IT ALL TOGETHER

- A 63 year old female is complaining of a sudden onset of chest pain and difficulty breathing. The patient's skin is cool and pale. Examination reveals a blood pressure of 60/40, respiratory rate of 24. The cardiac monitor displays a wide-complex tachycardia (QRS 0.16 sec) at 190 beats/minute.
- The patient has a past medical history of diabetes and heart disease and had a coronary bypass 3 1/2 years ago. Medications include Macrobid, Ibuprofen, Zantac and Micronase.
- You are instructed to administer 5 mg of Verapamil.
- Do you agree with this order? Why or why not?

## PUTTING IT ALL TOGETHER

The recommended compression to ventilation ratio in adult one-rescuer CPR is 15 compressions to 2 ventilations.

## PUTTING IT ALL TOGETHER

If atropine has proven unsuccessful and a pacemaker is not readily available, dopamine (or epinephrine) should be administered by continuous IV infusion.

## PUTTING IT ALL TOGETHER

- Airway management
  - Ventilation, oxygenation, intubation, suctioning
- External chest compressions
- Use of "quick-look" paddles and defibrillator
- Establishment of IV access and administration of drugs
- Placement of ECG electrodes
- Operation of the ECG machine
- Patient assessment
- Cardiac rhythm analysis
- Communication with base hospital (if prehospital personnel)

## PUTTING IT ALL TOGETHER

Pseudo-EMD is a term that refers to electrical activity associated with myocardial contractions too weak to produce a palpated or auscultated blood pressure.

## PUTTING IT ALL TOGETHER

- The patient is exhibiting signs and symptoms of congestive heart failure and possible myocardial infarction.
- Sit the patient up with legs dependent
- Administer oxygen and establish IV access.
- Pulse oximetry, 12-lead ECG, portable chest roentgenogram.
- Administer sublingual nitroglycerin and reassess.
- Administer furosemide 0.5-1.0 mg/kg IV bolus over 2 minutes
  - The patient regularly takes Lasix daily. The physician may elect to administer an initial dose of lasix that is double the normal daily oral dose.
- Consider morphine administration (1-3 mg) every 5 minutes titrated to effect.

## PUTTING IT ALL TOGETHER

- Despite the presence of a sinus tachycardia with PVCs on the monitor, the patient is pulseless and apneic. This situation is termed pulseless electrical activity.
- Initiate CPR. Administer high flow oxygen, insert an oropharyngeal airway and ventilate with a bag-valve device until the patient can be intubated.
- Establish two large bore IVs of normal saline or lactated Ringer's and infuse wide open.
- Consider treatable causes of this situation. Based on this patient's presentation, possible causes include hypovolemia (probable pelvic fracture), hypoxemia, cardiac tamponade.
- Consider use of the pneumatic anti-shock garment for temporary stabilization of the pelvic fracture.

## PUTTING IT ALL TOGETHER

- This patient is exhibiting signs of clinical instability as evidenced by the presence of chest pain, difficulty breathing and significant hypotension.
- Administer oxygen, establish IV access, administer sedation and countershock with 100 joules.
  - Wide-complex tachycardias associated with pulselessness, shock or congestive heart failure should always be presumed to be VT.
- Verapamil:
  - should not be administered to this patient because significant hypotension is present.
  - should not be administered to patients with a wide-complex tachycardia unless the tachycardia is known with certainty to be supraventricular in origin.

## PUTTING IT ALL TOGETHER

Immediate goals of postresuscitation care:

- Provide cardiorespiratory support to optimize tissue perfusion - especially to the brain.
- Transport the patient to the hospital emergency department and then to an appropriately equipped critical care unit.
- Attempt to identify the precipitating cause of the arrest.
- Initiate measures such as antidysrhythmic therapy to prevent recurrence.

## PUTTING IT ALL TOGETHER

- An 88 year old female states she feels her "heart is racing". This started about 1 1/2 hours ago while reading the newspaper. The patient's blood pressure is 128/90, respiratory rate 20. The patient denies chest pain or shortness of breath. The skin is warm, dry and pink. Breath sounds are clear.
- Her past medical history is significant for angina for which she takes Nitroglycerin as needed.
- How will you manage this patient?

Lead II

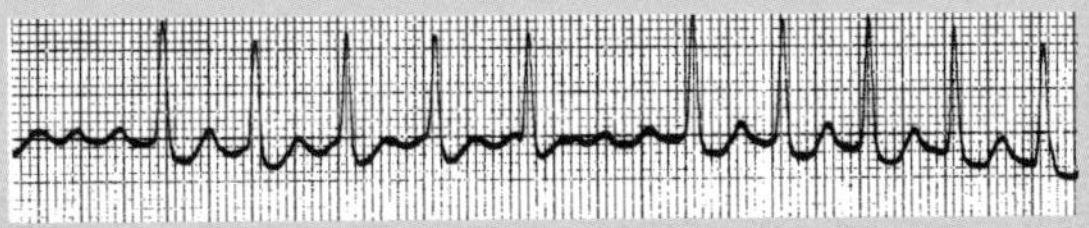

## PUTTING IT ALL TOGETHER

Name three signs and symptoms of a tension pneumothorax.

## PUTTING IT ALL TOGETHER

- An 80 year old female is found unconscious and unresponsive. Examination reveals a blood pressure of 110/80, respiratory rate of 24. The skin is warm and dry. There is no evidence of trauma. A neighbor states the patient is an insulin-dependent diabetic and has a history of hypertension.
- Medications include Tagamet, Isosorbide, Zaroxolyn, Lasix, Lanoxin and Indomethacin.
- A dextrostick reveals the patient's blood sugar to be between 20 and 40.
- How will you manage this patient?

Lead II

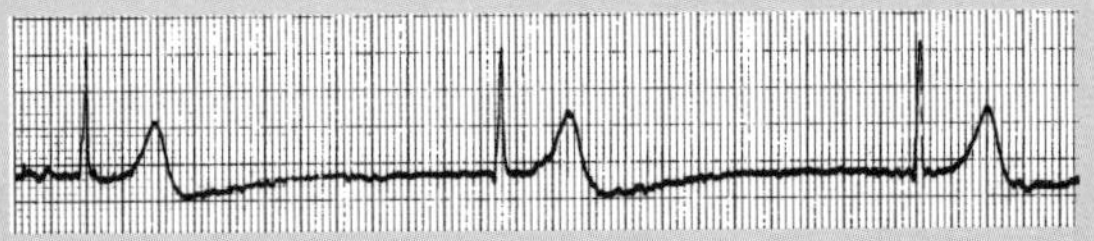

## PUTTING IT ALL TOGETHER

- A 64 year old male is complaining of severe chest pain, nausea and lightheadedness. His blood pressure is 76/42, respiratory rate 16. Breath sounds are clear. The patient states he was sitting outside in his lawn chair when his symptoms began. He takes no medications regularly and has no significant past medical history. The cardiac monitor reveals a complete (third-degree) AV block with a narrow-QRS at 44 beats per minute.
- How will you manage this patient?

## PUTTING IT ALL TOGETHER

- A 77 year old female is complaining of severe chest pain radiating across her chest and severe shortness of breath present for the past 2 1/2 hours. She is speaking in 2 word sentences and the presence of frothy sputum is noted. The patient appears to be in obvious distress. She is cyanotic and laboring to breath. Her respiratory rate is 32, pulse 80, blood pressure 130/70. Crackles are noted in all lung fields on auscultation.
- The patient has a past medical history of "heart problems" including a cardiac arrest 2 months ago. Medications include Lasix, Premarin, Cardizem, Ibuprofen and Lanoxin.
- As you continue your examination, the patient's respiratory rate decreases to 8 per minute and her blood pressure drops to 80/60. She is now unresponsive. The cardiac monitor reveals a sinus tachycardia at 128 per minute.
- How will you manage this patient?

## PUTTING IT ALL TOGETHER

Signs and symptoms of a tension pneumothorax include:
- hypotension
- tachycardia
- respiratory distress
- distended neck veins
    - may not be seen in the presence of hypovolemia
- tracheal deviation away from the affected side
    - a LATE sign
- hyperresonance to percussion on the affected side
- decreased or absent breath sounds on the affected side

## PUTTING IT ALL TOGETHER

- The rhythm shown is atrial flutter.
- Administer oxygen and establish IV access.
- This patient is clinically stable. Administer diltiazem (Cardizem) 0.25 mg/kg (approximately 20 mg) IV bolus over 2 minutes.
- Diltiazem may be repeated in 15 minutes if needed with 0.35 mg/kg (approximately 25 mg) IV bolus over 2 minutes.
    - Diltiazem may also be administered as a continuous IV infusion.
        - Mix 250 mg in 250 ml of IV solution.
        - The recommended initial infusion rate is 10 mg/hour.
- Other medications that may be considered include beta-blockers, verapamil, digoxin, procainamide, quinidine and anticoagulants.

## PUTTING IT ALL TOGETHER

- Administer oxygen and establish IV access.
- Pulse oximetry, 12-lead ECG, lab studies.
- Administer aspirin if no reason for exclusion.
- Medications for pain relief should be withheld until the patient's systolic BP is > 100 mm Hg.
- Atropine 0.5-1.0 mg may be administered RAPID IV bolus every 3-5 minutes to a maximum dose of 2-3 mg.
- Prepare for transcutaneous pacing.
- If these treatment measures are unsuccessful, a dopamine infusion (5-20 mcg/kg/min) may be administered.
- If evidence of thrombosis is present, evaluate the patient for possible thrombolytic therapy.

## PUTTING IT ALL TOGETHER

- Administer oxygen and establish IV access.
- The patient's blood sugar is between 20 and 40. Administer 50% dextrose and reassess.
- The patient's cardiac monitor reveals atrial fibrillation with a regular, bradycardic ventricular response. Draw lab studies to include a dig level.
- Pulse oximetry, 12-lead ECG, portable chest roentgenogram.
    - This patient woke up after administration of 50% dextrose. Lab studies revealed the patient's potassium level to be 1.7 (normal 3.5-4.5).

## PUTTING IT ALL TOGETHER

- Assist ventilations with a bag-valve device with 100% oxygen and intubate. Suction as needed.
- The question to be asked is, "Is this a rate problem, a pump problem or a volume problem"? Based on the patient's presenting signs and symptoms, this patient is experiencing a "pump problem" - acute pulmonary edema and acute myocardial infarction. Her signs and symptoms are consistent with cardiogenic shock.
- The patient's blood pressure is 80/60. First-line medications usually administered for acute pulmonary edema (nitroglycerin, furosemide, morphine) should be avoided as they may cause a further reduction in blood pressure. Dopamine is the drug of choice when the systolic BP is 70-100 mm Hg. Begin the infusion at 2.5 mcg/kg/minute and titrate, frequently reassessing the patient's condition.

# References


Aehlert, Barbara: *ACLS Quick Review Study Guide.* St. Louis: Mosby-Lifeline, 1994.

American Heart Association: *Textbook of Advanced Cardiac Life Support,* third edition, Dallas, 1987.

Bradshaw, Gordon VR: *Bradshaw's Blue Book, A Cross-Indexed Handbook of Over 1700 Prescription Drugs,* 1992.

Conover Mary B: *Understanding Electroardiography,* sixth edition. St. Louis: Mosby-Year Book, 1992.

Emergency Cardiac Care Committee and Subcommittees, American Heart Association: Guidelines for Cardiopulmonary Resuscitation and Emergency Cardiac Care. JAMA 268:2171-2295, 1992.

Flynn J, Bruce N: *Introduction to Critical Care Skills.* St. Louis: Mosby-Year Book, 1993.

Grauer K, Cavallaro DL: *ACLS: A Comprehensive Review - Volumes I and II,* third edition. St. Louis: Mosby-Year Book, 1993.

Marriott HJ, Conover MB: *Advanced Concepts in Arrhythmias,* second edition. St. Louis: Mosby-Year Book, 1988.

McKenry LM, Salerno E: *Mosby's Pharmacology in Nursing,* eighteenth edition. St. Louis: Mosby-Year Book, 1992.

Paraskos JA: Emergency Cardiac Care: The Science behind the Art. JAMA 268:2295-2297, 1992.

# Study Card Topics

## Airway Management

- Anatomy review
- Automatic transport ventilators
    - Advantages
- Bag-valve-device
    - Advantages
    - Common problems
    - Compliance
    - Features
    - Oxygen percentages
- Cricoid pressure
    - Purpose
    - Technique
- Endotracheal intubation
    - Advantages
    - Complications
    - Confirming tube placement
    - Equipment
    - Indications
    - Technique
    - Tube size
    - Use of stylet
- End-tidal CO2 detector
- Esophageal obturator airway
    - Contraindications
    - Equipment
- Foreign body airway obstruction
- Jaw thrust technique
- Minute volume
- Nasal cannula
    - Oxygen percentages
- Nasopharyngeal airway
    - Disadvantages
- Oropharyngeal airway
    - Advantages
    - Complications
    - Insertion
    - Sizing
- Pharyngotracheal lumen airway (PtLA)
    - Advantages
    - Contraindications
    - Disadvantages
    - Indications
- Pocket mask
    - Oxygen percentages
- Pulse oximetry
    - Advantages
    - Limitations
- Rescue breathing
- Respiratory distress
- Simple face mask
    - Oxygen flow rate
- Suctioning
    - Complications
    - Technique
- Surgical Cricothyroidotomy
    - Complications
    - Indications
    - Landmarks
- Tidal volume

## Dysrhythmia Recognition

- Action potential
- Analyzing a rhythm strip
- Anatomy review
- Automaticity
- AV junction
- Depolarization
- Dysrhythmias
    - Accelerated junctional rhythm
    - Agonal rhythm
    - Atrial fibrillation
    - Atrial flutter
    - AV blocks
        - First degree
        - Second-degree 2:1 conduction
        - Second-degree type I
        - Second-degree type II
        - Third-degree (complete)
    - Idioventricular rhythm
    - Junctional escape rhythm
    - Multifocal atrial tachycardia
    - Nonconducted premature atrial complexes
    - Premature atrial complexes
    - Premature junctional complexes
    - Premature ventricular complexes
        - Interpolated
        - R on T
        - Ventricular bigeminy
    - Sinus arrhythmia
    - Sinus tachycardia

## Electrical Therapy



## Myocardial Infarction

## Intravenous Techniques



## Pharmacology (Cardiovascular)

- Oxygen
  - Indications
- Procainamide
  - Indications
  - Precautions
- Sodium bicarbonate
  - Dosage
  - Indications
  - Precautions
- Sodium nitroprusside
  - Mechanism of action
  - Precautions
- Terminology Review
  - Chronotrope
  - Dromotrope
  - Inotrope
- Thrombolytic agents
  - Absolute contraindications
  - Complications
- Verapamil
  - Dosage
  - Indications
  - Mechanism of action

## Putting It All Together

- Acid-base balance
- Acute pulmonary edema
  - Management
- Asystole
  - Causes
  - Management
- Atrial fibrillation
  - Management
- Atrial flutter
  - Management
- Automatic chest compressor
  - Advantages
- Bradycardia
  - Management
  - Types
- Cardiogenic shock
  - Management
- Cardiopulmonary resuscitation
  - Complications
  - One-rescuer
  - Open-chest
  - Two-rescuer
- Critical incident debriefing
- Electrocution
  - Management
- Mechanical chest compressor
  - Advantages
- Near-drowning
  - Management
- Pneumatic anti-shock garment
  - Indications
- Postresuscitation management
- Pregnancy
  - Management
- Pseudo-EMD
- Pulseless electrical activity
  - Causes
  - Management
- Resuscitation team
  - Responsibilities
- Stroke
  - Management
  - Signs/symptoms
- Supraventricular tachycardia
  - Management
    - Stable
    - Unstable
- Tension pneumothorax
- Thrombolytic therapy
  - Door-to-drug interval
  - Qualifying criteria
- Ventricular fibrillation
  - Management
- Ventricular tachycardia
  - Management
    - Stable
- Volume problem
  - Management
- Wide-complex tachycardia
  - Management
    - Stable
  - Unstable

## Special Resuscitation Situations

- Electrocution
  - Factors determining impact of injuries
  - Management of cardiac arrest
  - Secondary injuries
  - Types of current
- Hypothermia
  - After-drop phenomenon
  - Basic life support management
  - Mild
  - Moderate
  - Severe